GETTING WELL NATURALLY SERIES

Premenstrual Syndrome

How You Can Benefit from Diet, Vitamins, Minerals, Herbs, Exercise, and Other Natural Methods

Michael T. Murray, N.D.

PRIMA PUBLISHING

PRIMA PUBLISHING and its colophon are registered trademarks of Prima Communications, Inc.

Warning—Disclaimer

Prima Publishing has designed this book to provide information in regard to the subject matter covered. It is sold with the understanding that the publisher and the author are not liable for the misconception or misuse of information provided. Every effort has been made to make this book as complete and as accurate as possible. The purpose of this book is to educate. The author and Prima Publishing shall have neither liability nor responsibility to any person or entity with respect to any loss, damage, or injury caused or alleged to be caused directly or indirectly by the information contained in this book. The information presented herein is in no way intended as a substitute for medical counseling.

Library of Congress Cataloging-in-Publication Data

Murray, Michael T.
    Premenstrual syndrome: how you can benefit from diet, vitamins, minerals, herbs, exercise, and other natural methods / Michael T. Murray.
        p.   cm.
    Includes bibliographical references and index.
    ISBN 0-7615-0820-1
    1. Premenstrual syndrome—Popular works.   2. Premenstrual syndrome—Alternative treatment.   I. Title.
RG165.M87   1997
618.1'72—dc21   97-5744
                                                                       CIP

97 98 99 00 01 HH 10 9 8 7 6 5 4 3 2 1
Printed in the United States of America

All products mentioned in this book are trademarks of their respective companies.

How to Order

Single copies may be ordered from Prima Publishing, P.O. Box 1260, Rocklin, CA 95677; telephone (916) 632-4400. Quantity discounts are also available. On your letterhead, include information concerning the intended use of the books and the number of books you wish to purchase.

Visit us online at http://www.primapublishing.com

Contents

Before You Read On

This book was written to empower you regarding your health care decisions; it is not designed to replace appropriate medical care. With that in mind, here are some important recommendations:

- Do not self-diagnose. Proper medical care is critical to good health. If you have symptoms suggestive of an illness, please consult a physician—preferably a naturopath, holistic physician or osteopath, chiropractor, or other natural health care specialist.

- If you are currently on a prescription medication, you absolutely must consult your doctor before discontinuing it. Furthermore, you must make your physician aware of all the nutritional supplements you are currently taking and why.

- If you wish to try a nutritional supplement as a therapeutic measure, discuss it with your physician. Since he or she is most likely unaware of the natural alternatives available, you may need to do some educating. Bring this book along with you to the doctor's office. The natural alternatives being recommended are based on published studies in medical journals. Key references are provided if your physician wants additional information.

- Remember, although many nutritional alternatives, such as nutritional supplements and planted-based medicines, are effective on their own, they work even better if they are part of a comprehensive natural treatment plan that focuses on diet and lifestyle.

About the Author

Michael T. Murray, N.D., is widely regarded as one of the world's leading authorities on natural medicine. He is a graduate, faculty member, and member of the Board of Trustees of Bastyr University in Seattle, Washington. In addition to maintaining a private medical practice, Dr. Murray is an accomplished writer, educator, and lecturer. He is the medical editor of *The American Journal of Natural Medicine*.

Dr. Murray serves on several editorial boards and advisory panels. As a consultant to the health food industry, Dr. Murray has been instrumental in bringing many effective natural products to America, including: ginkgo biloba extract, glucosamine sulfate, silymarin, enteric-coated peppermint oil, bilberry extract, DGL (deglycyrrhizinated licorice), saw palmetto berry extract, and the first thermogenic formula for weight loss.

1

An Overview of Premenstrual Syndrome

Premenstrual syndrome (PMS) is a major problem for many women. PMS is defined as a recurrent condition characterized by troublesome symptoms 7 to 14 days before menstruation.[1] Typical symptoms include decreased energy, tension, irritability, depression, headache, altered sex drive, breast pain, backache, abdominal bloating, and edema of the fingers and ankles. PMS is estimated to affect between 30% and 40% of menstruating women in the United States with peak occurrences among women in their thirties and forties. In most cases symptoms are relatively mild, however, in about 10% of all women symptoms can be quite severe. Severe PMS with depression, irritability, and extreme mood swings is referred to as *premenstrual dysphoric disorder.*[2]

Although PMS has been a well-defined clinical entity for over 60 years, many physicians argue that it does not really exist.[3] As a result, many women suffering from PMS do not receive proper treatment. Instead they are told that it is "all in your head." This view is gaining even more momentum because large pharmaceutical companies have recognized the huge market potential of women suffering from this syndrome and have begun to sponsor clinical trials using psychological drugs (e.g., antidepressant drugs such as Prozac and Zoloft, anti-anxiety drugs related to Valium, and gonadotropin-releasing hormone) to treat PMS symptoms. However the fact is that risks due to side effects of these drugs far outweigh their benefits.[4]

A more rational approach to the problem of PMS is identification of the causative factors and appropriate treatment using dietary therapy, nutritional supplementation, and exercise. Such an approach is provided in this book.

The Normal Menstrual Cycle

In order to understand the hormonal abnormalities that have been found in women with PMS, it is important to review the normal menstrual cycle. The menstrual cycle reflects the monthly rhythmic changes in the secretion rates of the female hormones and corresponding changes in the lining of the uterus and other female organs.

The menstrual cycle is controlled by the complex interactions of the hypothalamus, the pituitary gland, and the ovaries. Each month during the reproductive years, the secretion of various hormones is designed to accomplish two primary goals: (1) ensuring that only a single egg is released by the ovaries each month and (2) preparing the lining of the uterus, the endometrium, for implantation of the fertilized egg. To accomplish these goals, the concentrations of the primary female sexual hormones, estrogen and progesterone, fluctuate during the menstrual cycle.

The control center for the female hormonal system is the hypothalamus, a region of the brain roughly the size of a cherry, which is situated above the pituitary gland and below another area of the brain called the thalamus. The

Table 1.1   Signs and Symptoms of Premenstrual Syndrome

Behavioral	Female organs
Nervousness, anxiety, and irritability	Tender and enlarged breasts
Mood swings and mild to severe personality change	Uterine cramping
	Altered libido
Fatigue, lethargy, and depression	*General*
	Headache
Gastrointestinal	Backache
Abdominal bloating	Acne
Diarrhea and/or constipation	Edema of fingers and ankles
Change in appetite (usually craving of sugar)	

hypothalamus and pituitary gland are housed in the middle of the head just behind the eyes. The hypothalamus controls the female hormonal system by releasing hormones—e.g., gonadotropin-releasing hormone (GnRH) and follicle-stimulating hormone-releasing hormone (FSH-RH)—that stimulate the release of pituitary hormones.

In response to the hypothalamus, the pituitary gland releases follicle-stimulating hormone (FSH) and luteinizing hormone (LH). FSH is the hormone primarily responsible for the maturation of the egg (ovum) during the first phase of the menstrual cycle. FSH is called *follicle-stimulating hormone* because each egg within the ovary is housed inside individual follicles. LH is responsible for initiating ovulation—the release of the fully developed egg.

The release of LH is triggered by increasing estrogen levels as a result of the growing follicle. After ovulation, the eggless follicle is transformed into the corpus luteum, which functions primarily in the secretion of progesterone and estrogen with the goal being to help a fertilized egg become well-established in the uterine lining. If fertilization does not occur, the corpus luteum recedes, hormone production decreases, menses occurs approximately two weeks later, and the entire process begins anew.

The usual menstrual cycle is completed in about a month. It is divided into three phases: follicular, ovulatory, and luteal. The follicular phase lasts for 10 to 14 days; the ovulatory phase lasts for about 36 hours and involves the release of the egg; and the luteal phase lasts for about 14 days.

How Other Hormones Affect the Menstrual Cycle

Because of the complex interrelationships among the various components of the entire endocrine system, disorder of any of the individual members of the system (i.e., pituitary, ovaries, adrenals, thyroid, parathyroids, and pancreas) can lead to menstrual abnormalities and/or PMS. For example, low thyroid function (hypothyroidism) as well as elevated cortisol (an adrenal hormone) levels are very common in women with PMS and are discussed in Chapter 4 and Chapter 5, respectively. Prolactin (another hormone produced by the pituitary) often plays an important role in PMS and female infertility.

Prolactin's chief function is in the regulation of the mammary gland and milk secretion during and after pregnancy. Increased production of prolactin in lactating women can inhibit the maturation of the follicles in the ovary. In non-lactating women, elevated levels of prolactin are often linked to cases of PMS, menstrual abnormalities, absence of ovulation, ovarian cysts, and breast tenderness.

Hormonal Patterns in Women with PMS

Although there is a wide spectrum of symptoms, there are common hormonal patterns in PMS patients when compared to women who have no symptoms of PMS. The primary finding is that estrogen levels are elevated and plasma progesterone levels are reduced (or the ratio of estrogen to progesterone is increased) 5 to 10 days before the menses. In addition to this hormonal abnormality, hypothyroidism and/or elevated prolactin levels are common, FSH levels are typically elevated 6 to 9 days prior to the onset of menses, and aldosterone (a hormone produced by the adrenal glands that leads to sodium and water retention) levels are marginally elevated 2 to 8 days prior to the onset of menses.[1,5,6]

Corpus Luteum Insufficiency and PMS

PMS symptoms occur during the luteal phase of the menstrual cycle. This phase signifies the important role that the corpus luteum plays in the production of primarily progesterone, but also estrogen. It is theorized by many that PMS reflects *corpus luteum insufficiency*. Corpus luteum insufficiency is usually diagnosed by measuring the level of progesterone in the blood three weeks after onset of menstruation. If the level in the blood is below 10 to 12 mg per ml, corpus luteum insufficiency is a strong possibility.

In addition to PMS, corpus luteum insufficiency has also been linked to abnormal menstruation (excessive blood loss and absent, persistent, or more frequent menstruation), elevations in prolactin, and low thyroid function.[7]

Final Comments

PMS represents a *multifactorial* condition in that there is no single cause that explains PMS in every case. Many factors appear to play a role with some factors being more important in one case than another. Here is a brief list of the causative factors that will be examined more closely in this book:

Excess estrogen

Progesterone deficiency

Elevated prolactin levels

Nutritional factors

    Macronutrient disturbances/excesses

    Micronutrient deficiency

Hypothyroidism

Stress, endorphin deficiency, and adrenal dysfunction

Depression

The identification of the causes of PMS should be followed by appropriate therapy using natural measures to restore balance and harmony to the female hormonal system. Effective natural treatments are discussed in detail in throughout this book.

2

PMS Diagnosis and Classifications

Diagnosis of PMS is usually made by the association of the symptoms attributed to PMS with their occurrence during the luteal phase of the menstrual cycle. To aid in the diagnosis, symptom questionnaires are often used. Since recalled information is less accurate than immediate, in addition to a symptom questionnaire, it is a good idea to begin keeping a menstrual symptom diary. The diary will help in documenting improvement as well as further clarifying the symptom pattern. Both a questionnaire and sample diary are provided on page 9.

PMS Classifications

In an attempt to bring some order to the clinically and metabolically confusing picture of PMS, several experts have created classification systems that identify PMS sufferers into subgroups.[1] The system that I have the most experience with was developed by Dr. Guy Abraham and divides PMS into four distinct subgroups.[2] Each subgroup is linked to specific symptoms, hormonal patterns, and metabolic abnormalities. On page 9 is a menstrual symptom questionnaire based on Dr. Abraham's classifications, followed by a brief discussion of the individual subgroups. Please note that women rarely experience a particular subgroup in a pure form; usually there are aspects of two or more subgroups that a women with PMS experiences.

PMS-A

PMS-A (A = anxiety) is the most common symptom category and is found to be strongly associated with excessive estrogen and deficient progesterone during the premenstrual phase. Common symptoms in this category are anxiety, irritability, and emotional instability.

PMS-C

PMS-C (C = carbohydrate craving) is associated with increased appetite, craving for sweets, headaches, fatigue, fainting spells, and heart palpitations. Glucose tolerance tests (GTT) performed on PMS-C patients during the 5 to 10 days before their menses show a flattening of the early part of the curve (which usually implies excessive secretion of insulin in response to sugar consumption), whereas during other parts of the menstrual cycle their GTT is normal.[2] Currently, there is no clear explanation for this phenomenon, although an increased cellular capacity to bind insulin has been postulated. This increased binding capacity for insulin appears to be hormonally regulated, but other factors may also be involved such as a high salt intake or decreased magnesium or prostaglandin levels.

Menstrual Symptom Questionnaire

Date: _____

Grading of Symptoms

1 none
2 mild—present but does not interfere with activities
3 moderate—present and interferes with activities but not disabling
4 severe—disabling (unable to function)

Grade Your Symptoms for Last Menstrual Cycle Only

	Symptoms	Week After Period	Week Before Period
PMS-A	Nervous tension	_____	_____
	Mood swings	_____	_____
	Irritability	_____	_____
	Anxiety	_____	_____
		TOTAL _____	TOTAL _____
PMS-H	Weight gain	_____	_____
	Swelling of extremities	_____	_____
	Breast tenderness	_____	_____
	Abdominal bloating	_____	_____
		TOTAL _____	TOTAL _____
PMS-C	Headache	_____	_____
	Craving for sweets	_____	_____
	Increased appetite	_____	_____
	Heart pounding	_____	_____
	Fatigue	_____	_____
	Dizziness or fainting	_____	_____
		TOTAL _____	TOTAL _____
PMS-D	Depression	_____	_____
	Forgetfulness	_____	_____
	Crying	_____	_____
	Confusion	_____	_____
	Insomnia	_____	_____
		TOTAL _____	TOTAL _____
	Total MSQ score	_____	_____

Other symptoms

	Oily skin	_____	_____
	Acne	_____	_____

During first two days of periods

	Menstrual cramps	_____
	Menstrual backache	_____

PMS-D

PMS-D (D = depression) is the least common and is relatively rare in its pure form. Its key symptom is depression, which is usually associated with low levels of neurotransmitters in the central nervous system. In PMS-D patients this is most likely due to increased breakdown of the neurotransmitters as a result of decreased levels of estrogen (in contrast to PMS-A, which shows just the opposite results). The decreased ovarian estrogen output has been attributed to a stress-induced increase in adrenal androgen and/or progesterone secretion.

PMS-H

PMS-H (H = hyperhydration) is characterized by weight gain (greater than three pounds), abdominal bloating and discomfort, breast tenderness, congestion, and occasional swelling of the face, hands, and ankles. These symptoms are due to an increased fluid volume secondary to an excess of the hormone aldosterone, which causes increased fluid retention. Aldosterone excess during the premenstrual phase of PMS-H patients may arise due to stress, estrogen excess, magnesium deficiency, or excess salt intake.

An Alternative Classification System

Abraham's system is very useful in quickly identifying possible causes in a given case of PMS. However, I prefer to classify my patients according to the causative factor. In order to classify the patient, I must first uncover the causative factor(s). Again, the most common causative factors are:

Excess estrogen
Progesterone deficiency
Elevated prolactin levels
Nutritional factors
    Macronutrient disturbances/excesses
    Micronutrient deficiency
Hypothyroidism
Stress, endorphin deficiency, and adrenal dysfunction
Depression

The detection of these causative factors involves a diagnostic hierarchy based upon the patient's clinical picture and history. Following the steps listed below should lead to the proper identification of the causative factor. As a result, a more effective treatment plan can be tailored to the specific needs of the individual and, as a result, better relief can be achieved.

Detecting Causal Factors

1. Begin following the recommendations summarized in Chapter 11.

2. Determine your basal body temperature (discussed in Chapter 4, page 31). If your basal body temperature is below 97.8 degrees Fahrenheit or if you are suffering from other symptoms associated with thyroid-affected PMS, consult your physician for complete thyroid function testing (discussed in Chapter 4).

3. Determine if depression may be a factor by taking the self-test in Chapter 6 (page 49). If it is, follow the recommendations given in Chapter 6.

4. If you have followed the recommendations in Chapter 11, ruled out or addressed hypothyroidism or

depression, and have not improved after three months, ask your physician to perform a complete blood count and chemistry panel (including serum ferritin, thyroid panel, and estrogen, progesterone, and prolactin levels) on day 21 of your cycle. (Day 21 of your cycle is the twenty-first day after you begin bleeding.) The test should include:

Complete blood count
  White blood cell count
  Red blood cell count
  Hemoglobin
  Mean corpuscular volume
  Mean corpuscular hemoglobin
  Mean corpuscular hemoglobin concentration
  Platelet count
  Differential
    Neutrophils
    Lymphocytes
    Monocytes
    Eosinophils

Chemistry Panel
  Sodium
  Potassium
  Chloride
  CO_2
  Anion gap
  Protein
  Albumin
  Globulin
  A/G ratio
  LDH

AST (SGOT)

ALT (SGPT)

Bilirubin

   Total

   Direct

Alkaline phosphatase

Calcium

Phosphorus

Uric acid

BUN/Creatinine

Glucose

Cholesterol

Triglycerides

Thyroid panel

   T3 uptake

   Thyroxine

   Free thyroxine index

Ferritin

Progesterone

Estrogen

5. If there are no apparent abnormalities in the complete blood count and chemistry panel, additional tests I may recommend include liver detoxification profile (see Chapter 3, page 24), adrenal stress index (see Chapter 5, page 38), and food allergy panel (see Chapter 7, page 103).

Final Comments

Working with a physician knowledgeable about nutritional therapy can be of great benefit. If you need help finding a nutritionally oriented physician in your area who may be familiar with the recommendations in this book, contact the following organizations:

The American Association of Naturopathic Physicians
P.O. Box 20386
Seattle, WA 98102
(206) 323-7610

The American Holistic Medical Association
4101 Lake Boone Trail, #201
Raleigh, NC 26707
(919) 787-5146

American College of Advancement in Medicine (ACAM)
23121 Verdugo Drive, Suite 204
Laguna Hills, CA, 92653
1-800-532-3688 (outside California) or 1-800-435-6199 (inside California)

3

The Estrogen to Progesterone Ratio

One of the most common findings in women with PMS is an elevated estrogen to progesterone ratio.[1-6] Most commonly this derangement is caused by a combination of mild estrogen excess and mild progesterone deficiency. An increased estrogen to progesterone ratio contributes to PMS by leading to:

Impaired liver function

Reduced manufacture of serotonin

Decreased action of vitamin B_6

Increased aldosterone secretion

Increased prolactin secretion

Estrogen Excess and Liver Function

In the early 1940s, Dr. Morton Biskind observed an apparent relationship between B-vitamin deficiency and PMS.[7,8]

Table 3.1   Causes of Cholestasis

Estrogen excess or birth control pills
Pregnancy
Presence of gallstones
Alcohol
Endotoxins
Hereditary disorders such as Gilbert's syndrome
Anabolic steroids
Common chemicals such as pesticides, herbicides, and solvents
Acetaminophen

He postulated that PMS, as well as excessive menstruation and fibrocystic breast disease, was due to an excess in estrogen levels caused by decreased detoxification and elimination by the liver due to vitamin-B deficiency. There appears to be support for Dr. Biskind's theory.

The liver utilizes various B vitamins to detoxify estrogen and excrete it in the bile. Estrogen excess is known to produce what is known medically as *cholestasis,* which signifies diminished bile flow or stasis of bile. Naturopathic physicians often refer to this condition as a "sluggish liver." It reflects minimal impairment of liver function because normal indicators of liver function, such as liver enzymes (alkaline phosphatase, SGOT, SGPT, and GGTP), are not elevated. However, because of the liver's important role in numerous metabolic processes, even minor impairment of liver function can have profound effects.

Cholestasis can be caused by a great number of factors besides estrogen excess (see Table 3.1 above). The presence of cholestasis may be a predisposing factor to PMS because with cholestasis there is reduced estrogen detoxification and clearance. Hence, a positive-feedback scenario is produced.

Many American women suffer from cholestasis, which is indicated by the tremendous frequency of gallstones in this population. Nearly 20% of the U.S. female and 8% of the U.S. male population over the age of 40 are found to have gallstones on biopsy. In the United States, approximately 500,000 gallbladders are removed each year because of gallstones. The prevalence of gallstones in this country has been related to the high-fat/low-fiber diet consumed by the majority of Americans.

Effects of Estrogen on Neurotransmitters

Another possible result of the increase in the estrogen to progesterone ratio is impairment of neurotransmitter synthesis and endorphin activity. Neurotransmitters are compounds that transmit the nerve impulse. A group of neurotransmitters known as *monoamines* are made from dietary amino acids—the building block molecules of proteins. For example, the amino acid *tryptophan* serves as the precursor to serotonin and melatonin while the amino acids *phenylalanine* and *tyrosine* are precursors to dopamine, epinephrine, and norepinephrine.

According to the dominant medical view, depression is characterized by imbalances of monoamines. In addition to estrogen-induced alterations, environmental, nutritional, psychological, and genetic factors can lead to an imbalance in monoamines that might result in depression. Antidepressant drugs act by increasing different monoamines in the brain by blocking the re-uptake, blocking the breakdown, or enhancing the effect of a specific monoamine. Antidepressant drug therapy for PMS is gaining increased popularity among many M.D.s; however, these drugs have side effects and do not address the basic cause. There are more appropriate ways to address the alterations in neurotransmitters and chief among them is normalizing estrogen to progesterone ratios. The majority of the over 12 million patients on Prozac are women between the ages of 25 and 50. This is the same population that has a high frequency of PMS. Alternatives to Prozac and other antidepressant drugs are given in Chapter 6.

Estrogen Excess and Endorphin Levels

Estrogen excess during the luteal phase also negatively affects endorphin levels. Endorphins are the body's own mood-elevating and pain-relieving substances. One study found a direct correlation between an increased estrogen to progesterone ratio and endorphin activity in the brain.[3] In essence, when the estrogen to progesterone ratio was increased there was a decline in endorphin levels. This reduction is significant considering the known ability of endorphins to normalize or improve mood. Other studies have shown that low endorphin levels during the luteal phase are common in women with PMS.[9] Endorphins are lowered by stress and raised by exercise. The role of endorphins is further discussed in Chapter 5.

Estrogen Impairs Vitamin B$_6$

The way in which estrogen excess during the luteal phase negatively affects neurotransmitter and endorphin levels may be secondary to impairment of vitamin B$_6$ action. Vitamin B$_6$ (pyridoxine) is an extremely important B vitamin involved in the formation of body proteins, structural compounds, chemical transmitters in the nervous system, red blood cells, and hormonelike compounds known as *prostaglandins*. Vitamin B$_6$ is critical to maintaining hormonal balance.

It is well-known that estrogens negatively affect vitamin B_6 function. Vitamin B_6 levels are typically quite low in depressed patients, especially women taking estrogens (birth control pills or Premarin).[10,11] Vitamin B_6 supplementation has been shown to exert positive effects on PMS symptoms (particularly depression) in many women (this is discussed in greater detail in Chapter 8, page 106). The improvement is achieved via a combined reduction in mid-luteal estrogen levels and an increase in mid-luteal progesterone levels.

Estrogen's Effects on Aldosterone

As stated previously, aldosterone is a hormone produced by the adrenal glands which leads to sodium and water retention. In many cases of PMS, aldosterone levels are marginally elevated 2 to 8 days prior to the onset of menses. This elevation may be a result of estrogen excess increasing the secretion of aldosterone.

Estrogen and Prolactin Secretion

Excessive levels of prolactin are implicated in many cases of PMS, especially in women experiencing breast pain or fibrocystic breast disease (discussed in Chapter 10).[12,13] Estrogens, both internally produced and ingested as birth control pills or Premarin, are known to increase prolactin secretion by the pituitary gland. Following the recommendations given below for lowering the luteal-phase estrogen to progesterone ratio may be all that is necessary to lower prolactin levels. In particular, the herb *Vitex agnus-castus* (chaste berry) may prove to be very useful in cases of high prolactin levels due to corpus-luteum insufficiency (discussed in Chapter 9, page 129). Vitamin B_6 and zinc supplementation also lower prolactin levels and are discussed in Chapter 8. Prolactin levels also tend to be elevated in low thyroid function.

Reducing the Estrogen to Progesterone Ratio Naturally

Central to effective treatment in most cases of PMS is lowering the luteal-phase estrogen to progesterone ratio. An elevation in this ratio may be the underlying factor in the hormonal, neurotransmitter, endorphin, and other physiological disturbances in most cases of PMS. Effective treatment usually involves the following steps:

Improving Your Diet

A number of dietary factors are known to reduce circulating estrogens or block the attachment of estrogen to receptor sites. Chief among these dietary recommendations are increasing your consumption of plant foods (vegetables, fruits, legumes, whole grains, nuts, and seeds); lowering or eliminating your consumption of meat and dairy; reducing your fat and sugar intake; and increasing your consumption of soy foods. These dietary recommendations are discussed in detail in Chapter 7. In addition, it is important to reduce the load of environmental estrogens in your diet by avoiding foods sprayed with pesticides and herbicides.

Establishing Proper Gastrointestinal Flora

One of the key ways in which the liver detoxifies cancer-causing chemicals, as well as hormones such as estrogen, is by attaching glucuronic acid to the toxin and excreting it in the bile. Beta-glucuronidase is a bacterial enzyme that uncouples (breaks) the bond between excreted toxins and glucuronic acid. Excess beta-glucuronidase activity is associated with an increased cancer risk, particularly estrogen-dependent breast cancer, and presumably PMS. The activity of this enzyme can be reduced by establishing a proper bacterial flora.[14] Following the dietary guidelines in Chapter 7 goes a long way toward achieving this goal. In addition, initial supplementation with probiotics can be effective. *Probiotics* literally translated means "for life," a term used to signify the health-promoting effects of these "friendly bacteria." The most important friendly bacteria are *Lactobacillus acidophilus* and *Bifidobacterium bifidum*.

The dosage of a commercial probiotic supplement is based upon the number of live organisms. The ingestion of 1 to 10 billion viable *L. acidophilus* or *B. bifidum* cells daily is a sufficient dosage for most people. Amounts exceeding this may induce mild gastrointestinal disturbances, while smaller amounts may not be able to colonize the gastrointestinal tract. Probiotics are extremely safe and are not associated with any side effects.

In order to provide benefit, products containing *L. acidophilus* and *B. bifidum* must provide live organisms in such a manner that they survive the hostile environment of the gastrointestinal tract. Several factors—such as species, strain, adherence, growth media, and diet—are involved in successful colonization. Typically, a high-quality commercial preparation will produce greater colonization than simply eating yogurt. One of the key reasons is that yogurt is usually made with *L. bulgaricus* or *Streptococcus thermophilus*. While these two bacteria are friendly and possess some health benefits, they are only transient visitors to the gastrointestinal tract and do not colonize the colon.

Proper manufacturing, packaging, and storing of the probiotic is necessary to ensure viability, the right amount of moisture, and freedom from contamination. Lactobacilli do not respond well to freeze-drying (lyophilization), spray drying, or conventional frozen storage. Excessive temperatures during packaging or storage can dramatically reduce viability. Also, unless the product has been shown to be stable, refrigeration is necessary. Some products do not have to be refrigerated until after the bottle has been opened.

While a number of excellent companies provide high-quality probiotic products, it is difficult to sort through all of the manufacturer's claims of superiority, and unfortunately some products have been shown to contain no active *L. acidophilus*. In fact, one study conducted at the University of Washington concluded, "Most of the lactobacilli-containing products currently available [1990] either do not contain the *Lactobacillus* species advertised and/or contain other bacteria of questionable benefit."[15]

I feel confident recommending products that have been developed by Professor Khem M. Shahani, Ph.D., of the University of Nebraska. Dr. Shahani is considered the world's foremost expert on probiotics and is the developer of the DDS-1 strain of *L. acidophilus*—often referred to as the "super-strain" because it exerts benefits far greater than those of the other (more than 200) strains of *L. acidophilus*. The author of over 190 scientific studies on the role of lactobacilli in human health, Dr. Shahani has personally endorsed several products available in health food stores.

Supplementing with Vitamins and Minerals

Estrogen excess is known to increase nutritional needs for B vitamins, magnesium, and possibly other nutrients. In addition, B vitamins and magnesium are necessary for the proper detoxification of estrogens. Follow the guidelines for nutritional supplementation given in Chapter 8.

Enhancing Liver Detoxification

It is amazing how well the liver survives the constant onslaught of toxic chemicals that it is responsible for detoxifying. Every effort should be made to promote optimal liver function in women with PMS. In particular, it is important to support the liver's ability to detoxify not only estrogen but also the various herbicides and pesticides which exert estrogenic activity including DDT, dioxin, 2,4,5-T, 2,4-D, and the halogenated compounds PCB and PCP. These chemicals are discussed in greater detail in Chapter 7; I believe they may be playing a factor in the increasing rates of PMS and breast cancer in American women.

Supporting liver function focuses on protecting the liver by following the dietary guidelines given in Chapter 7 and the nutritional supplement recommendations given in Chapter 8. In addition, naturopathic physicians often use formulas containing *lipotropic factors*. Lipotropic factors are substances that hasten the removal or decrease the deposition of fat and bile in the liver through their interaction with fat metabolism. In essence, they produce a decongestant effect on the liver and promote improved liver function and fat metabolism. Compounds commonly employed as lipotropic agents include choline, methionine, betaine, folic acid, and vitamin B_{12}, along with herbs that increase the flow of bile (choleretics) or cause the gallbladder to contract (cholagogues). Most major manufacturers of nutritional supplements offer lipotropic formulas. When taking a lipotropic formula it is essential to take enough of the formula to provide a daily dose of 1,000 mg of choline and 500 mg of methionine and/or cysteine.

If a woman with PMS does not respond to typical recommendations after three months, it is likely that there is disruption of her liver's normal detoxification pathways. A liver detoxification profile can be invaluable in providing this information. This laboratory test is designed to assess the liver's ability to detoxify different chemicals. The test involves analyzing saliva samples following the ingestion of a premeasured amount of caffeine and urine samples after the ingestion of acetaminophen (Tylenol) and aspirin. The liver's ability to detoxify these compounds will be apparent based on the metabolites produced in the saliva and urine.

Laboratories that I am familiar with which provide a liver detoxification profile are Great Smokies Diagnostic Laboratory (1-800-522-4762), National BioTech Laboratory (1-800-846-6285), Diagnos-Techs (1-800-87-TESTS), and Meridian Valley Clinical Laboratory (1-206-859-8700). All of these laboratories provide general guidelines for addressing the abnormalities noted.

Using Herbs

Chaste berry (*Vitex agnus-castus*) and phytoestrogen-containing herbs such as dong quai, black cohosh, and licorice are popular herbal recommendations for PMS. Their appropriate use is described in detail in Chapter 9. For most cases I tend to recommend chaste berry. It is particularly useful in corpus luteum insufficiency and/or elevated prolactin levels. The usual dosage of chaste berry extract (often standardized to contain 0.5% agnuside) is 175 to 225 mg daily.

Final Comments

You may be asking, "If one of the primary features of PMS for most women is an elevated estrogen to progesterone ratio, why not simply take progesterone?" Although progesterone administration is a popular recommendation made by many physicians (M.D.s and N.D.s, alike), I have some reservations. First of all, although progesterone administration has been the most common prescription for PMS by the medical community, controlled clinical trials have failed to consistently demonstrate the superiority of progesterone therapy over a placebo (there is a significant placebo response in PMS, by the way).[16-19] The studies that are positive have used dosages (200 mg to 400 mg twice daily as a vaginal or rectal suppository from 14 days before the expected onset of menstruation until the onset of vaginal bleeding) that far exceed the normal levels for progesterone and the estrogen to progesterone ratio.[20,21] Side effects of progesterone administration, although generally mild, are common. In a recent double-blind study that did show a positive effect with progesterone therapy (400 mg twice a day by vaginal or rectal administration), adverse events were reported by 51% of patients in the progesterone treatment group (compared to 43% in the placebo group).[21] Irregularity of menstruation, vaginal itching, and headaches were reported more frequently by the women taking the progesterone. Second, I would rather help the body *naturally* improve the estrogen and progesterone ratio by addressing the underlying causative factors rather than artificially and drastically tipping the ratio in favor of progesterone.

I cannot in good conscience recommend unsupervised use of progesterone creams for treating PMS. However, I realize that progesterone creams are being promoted and used out in the marketplace. Here are some guidelines if you elect to give a progesterone-containing cream a try.

First of all, make sure that the level (in milligrams) of progesterone per dosage unit is provided so that you can calculate how much of the cream is required to achieve the high dosage required (200 mg to 400 mg applied twice daily intra-vaginally). A distinction must be made between prescription progesterone preparations and some of the over-the-counter progesterone-containing creams, including those misrepresented as "yam concentrates." Mexican yam is a source of a compound known as *diosgenin* that can be converted in a laboratory environment to progesterone as well as the hormone DHEA (dehydroepiandrosterone). There is no evidence that such a conversion occurs in the human body. Buyer beware. Some companies label a progesterone-containing cream as a yam concentrate as a marketing ploy while other companies market a true yam concentrate without any significant levels of progesterone as providing the same benefit as a progesterone-containing cream. In both cases this misrepresentation is wrong.

Second, intravaginal administration is more effective than simply applying the cream to anywhere on the skin. In fact, progesterone applied to the skin (non-mucous membranes) is poorly absorbed.

Finally, monitor your progesterone levels by ordering a saliva test for progesterone by contacting Aeron Life Cycles Laboratories (1-800-631-7900) after one month of use and adjust your dosage accordingly.

4

Low Thyroid Function in PMS

Low thyroid function (hypothyroidism) has been shown to affect a large percentage of women with PMS. For example, in one study published in the prestigious *New England Journal of Medicine,* 51 out of 54 PMS subjects demonstrated low thyroid status compared to 0 out of 12 for the control group.[1] In another study, it was 7 out of 10 in the PMS group and 0 out of 9 for the control group.[2] Other studies have only shown hypothyroidism to be slightly more common in women with PMS compared to controls.[3,4] The bottom line is that many women with PMS and confirmed hypothyroidism who are given thyroid hormone experience complete relief of symptoms.[1]

Hypothyroidism Is Common in Women

In general it can be stated that hypothyroidism is common in women; current estimates indicate that nearly 20% (one out of five women) in the United States have hypothyroidism. These estimates are based largely on using altered levels of thyroid hormones in the blood, namely, low levels of thyroxine and T3-uptake and an increased level of thyroid-stimulating hormone (TSH). However, it is now known that standard thyroid blood tests are not sensitive enough to diagnose milder forms of hypothyroidism. As a result, many people with mild hypothyroidism are going undiagnosed.

The best diagnostic measures to undercover many cases of mild hypothyroidism are the thyroid stimulation test and basal body temperature. Both of these procedures are discussed below.

The Importance of Ruling Out Hypothyroidism

Undiagnosed hypothyroidism is a serious concern because failure to treat an underlying condition such as hypo-thyroidism will reduce the effectiveness of nutritional therapies for PMS and other conditions.

Since the hormones of the thyroid gland regulate metabolism in every cell of the body, a deficiency of thyroid hormones can affect virtually all body functions. The severity of symptoms in adults ranges from extremely mild deficiencies, which are barely detectable (subclinical hypothyroidism), to severe, life-threatening deficiencies, (myxedema).

Manifestations of Adult Hypothyroidism

Since thyroid hormone affects every cell of the body, a deficiency will usually result in a large number of signs and symptoms. A brief review of the common manifestations of hypothyroidism on several body systems is given below.

Metabolic

The metabolic manifestations of hypothyroidism reflect a general decrease in the rate of utilization of fat, protein, and carbohydrates. Moderate weight gain combined with cold intolerance is a common finding. Cholesterol and triglyceride levels are increased in even the mildest forms of hypothyroidism.[5] This elevation greatly increases the risk of serious cardiovascular disease. Studies have shown an increased rate of heart disease due to atherosclerosis in individuals with hypothyroidism.[6,7]

Hypothyroidism also leads to increased capillary permeability and slow lymphatic drainage. Often this will result in swelling of tissue (edema).

Endocrine

A variety of hormonal symptoms can exist in hypothyroidism. Perhaps the most common is a loss of libido (sexual drive) in men and menstrual abnormalities in women.

Women with mild hypothyroidism have prolonged and heavy menstrual bleeding, with a shorter menstrual cycle (time from the start of one period to the next). Infertility may also be a problem. If the hypothyroid woman does become pregnant, miscarriages, premature deliveries, and stillbirths are common. Rarely does a pregnancy terminate in normal labor and delivery in the hypothyroid woman.

Skin, Hair, and Nails

Dry, rough skin covered with fine superficial scales is seen in most hypothyroid individuals; the hair is coarse, dry, and brittle. Hair loss can be quite severe. The nails become thin and brittle and typically show transverse grooves.

Psychological

The brain appears to be quite sensitive to low levels of thyroid hormone. Depression along with weakness and fatigue are usually the first symptoms of hypothyroidism.[8,9] Later the hypothyroid individual may have difficulty concentrating and be extremely forgetful.

Muscular and Skeletal

Muscle weakness and joint stiffness is a predominant feature of hypothyroidism.[10] Some individuals with hypothyroidism may also experience muscle and joint pain and tenderness.[11]

Cardiovascular

Hypothyroidism is thought to predispose one to atherosclerosis due to the increase in cholesterol and triglycerides in one's body.[9-11] Hypothyroidism can also cause hypertension, reduce the function of the heart, and reduce heart rate.

Other Manifestations

Shortness of breath, constipation, and impaired kidney function are some of the other common features of hypothyroidism.[12]

Diagnosing Hypothyroidism

The routine diagnosis of hypothyroidism involves measuring levels of thyroid hormones in the blood. Low levels of thyroxine and T3-uptake and an increased level of thyroid-stimulating hormone (TSH) are usually definitive for hypothyroidism. However, as stated above, in milder cases of thyroid hormone insufficiency, the usual thyroid hormone values may be in the normal range. The TRH stimulation test and the basal body temperature test are often used to detect hypothyroidism when the usual thyroid hormone measurements come back normal.

The TRH stimulation test involves determining the level of TSH prior to and after the administration of an intravenous injection of synthetic thyrotropin-releasing hormone (TRH). In patients with hypothyroidism there will either be an increase or a decrease in the normal response to TRH depending upon whether the hypothyroidism is due to a problem with the thyroid gland or pituitary, respectively.

Obviously, you cannot perform the TRH stimulation test at home, but there is another functional test that you can do yourself—determining your basal body temperature. Your body temperature reflects your metabolic rate, which is largely determined by hormones secreted by the thyroid gland. Therefore, the function of your thyroid gland can be determined by simply measuring your basal body temperature, which is your body temperature at rest. Several authors have proposed that the basal body temperature is perhaps the most sensitive functional test of thyroid function.[12,13] A simple method for taking your basal body temperature is detailed below. All that is needed is a thermometer.

How to Take Your Basal Body Temperature

1. Shake down the thermometer to below 95 degrees Fahrenheit and place it by your bed before going to sleep at night.

2. On waking, place the thermometer in your armpit for a full 10 minutes. It is important to make as little

movement as possible. Lying and resting with your eyes closed is best. Do not get up until the 10-minute test is completed.

3. After 10 minutes, read and record the temperature and date.

4. Record the temperature for at least three mornings (preferably at the same time of day) and give the information to your physician. Menstruating women must perform the test on the second, third, and fourth days of menstruation. Men and postmenopausal women can perform the test at any time.

Interpretation Your basal body temperature should be between 97.8 and 98.2 degrees Fahrenheit. Lower basal body temperatures may reflect hypothyroidism. Common signs and symptoms of hypothyroidism are low basal body temperature, depression, difficulty in losing weight, dry skin, headaches, lethargy or fatigue, menstrual problems, recurrent infections, constipation, and sensitivity to cold.

High basal body temperatures (above 98.6 degrees Fahrenheit) are less common, but may be evidence of hyperthyroidism. Common signs and symptoms of hyperthyroidism include bulging eyeballs, fast pulse, hyperactivity, inability to gain weight, insomnia, irritability, menstrual problems, and nervousness.

Correcting Hypothyroidism

The medical treatment of hypothyroidism, in all but its mildest forms, involves the use of desiccated (freeze-dried) whole thyroid or synthetic versions of the thyroid hormones (e.g., Synthroid), both of which are available only by prescription. Although synthetic versions of thyroxine (T4) have become popular, many physicians (particularly naturopathic physicians) still prefer the use of desiccated natural thyroid, which is complete with all thyroid hormones, including thyroxine and T3. At this time, it appears that thyroid hormone replacement *is* necessary in the majority of people with hypothyroidism.

The thyroid extracts sold in health food stores are required by the Food and Drug Administration (FDA) to be thyroxine-free. However, it is nearly impossible to remove all the hormone from the gland. In other words, think of thyroid preparations that you can obtain at the health food store as milder forms of desiccated natural thyroid. If you have mild hypothyroidism, these preparations may provide enough support to help you with your thyroid problem.

Because it is important to nutritionally support the thyroid gland by ensuring adequate intake of key nutrients required in the manufacture of thyroid hormone, most thyroid products available at health food stores also contain supportive nutrients such as iodine, zinc, and tyrosine.

Nutritional Support in Hypothyroidism

The manufacture of thyroid hormones within the thyroid gland is dependent on several important nutrients. Deficiency of any of a number of vitamins and minerals, especially iodine, or even ingestion of certain foods, can result in hypothyroidism.

Iodine Thyroid hormones are made from iodine and the amino acid tyrosine. The recommended dietary allowance (RDA) for iodine in adults is quite small, 150 micrograms (mcg). The average intake of iodine in the United States is estimated to be over 600 mcg per day. Too much iodine can actually inhibit the thyroid gland. For this reason and because the only function of iodine in the body is for thyroid hormone synthesis, it is recommended that dietary levels or supplementation of iodine not exceed 600 mcg per day for any length of time.

Goitrogens   Some foods contain substances that prevent the utilization of iodine. These foods are termed *goitrogens* and include such foods as turnips, cabbage, mustard, cassava root, soybeans, peanuts, pine nuts, and millet. Cooking usually inactivates goitrogens.

Vitamins and Minerals   Zinc, vitamin E, and vitamin A function together in many body processes including the manufacture of thyroid hormone.[14] A deficiency of any of these nutrients results in lower levels of active thyroid hormone. Low zinc levels are common in the elderly as is hypothyroidism.[15] There may be a correlation.

The B vitamins riboflavin (B2), niacin (B3), and pyridoxine (B6), as well as vitamin C, are also necessary for normal thyroid hormone manufacture.[16]

Final Comments

Another recommendation to improve thyroid function is to engage in regular exercise. Exercise is known to stimulate thyroid gland secretion and increase tissue sensitivity to thyroid hormone.[16] Many of the health benefits of exercise may be a result of improved thyroid function. The health benefits of exercise are especially significant in overweight hypothyroid individuals who are dieting (restricting their food intake in order to lose weight). A consistent effect of dieting is a decrease in the metabolic rate as the body strives to conserve fuel. Exercise has been shown to prevent this decline in metabolic rate.[16]

5

Stress, Endorphins, and Exercise

Like many common conditions associated with modern living, stress definitely plays a role in PMS. When stress is extreme, unusual, or long-lasting it triggers biological changes in the brain largely as a result of altered adrenal gland function and endorphin secretion or action. These changes produce a domino effect as they lead to alterations in normal physiology. Effective treatment of PMS must include stress management.

Assessing Stress

Stress is a major factor to consider in the individual with PMS. To determine the role that stress may play, I rely a lot on my clinical judgment. I also utilize a popular method of rating stress levels—the Social Readjustment Rating Scale (see Table 5.1) developed by Holmes and Rahe.[1] The scale was originally designed to predict the likelihood of a person getting a serious disease due to stress. Various life-change events are numerically rated according to their potential for causing disease. Notice that even events commonly viewed as positive, such as an outstanding personal achievement, carry with them stress.

Interpreting Your Score

The standard interpretation of the Social Readjustment Rating Scale is that a total of 200 or more units in one year is considered to be predictive of the likelihood of getting a serious disease. However, rather than using the scale solely to predict the likelihood of the patient getting a serious disease, I utilize the scale as an opportunity to gain insight into a person's stress level. Not everyone reacts to stressful events in the same way, thus, I utilize the scale as a rough indicator of a person's stress level.

Stress and the Adrenal Glands

To a very large extent the ability to withstand stress involves healthy adrenal gland function. These glands lie just above the kidneys and are responsible for secreting an important group of hormones called *corticosteroids.* The three major types of corticosteroids are glucocorticoids, mineralcorticoids, and 17-ketosteroids (sex hormones).

The glucocorticoids—mainly cortisol, corticosterone, and cortisone—exert a profound effect upon the metabolism of glucose. These hormones increase serum glucose. In addition, glucocorticoids reduce inflammation and the allergic response.

The mineralcorticoids, of which aldosterone is the most important, have profound effects on minerals. Specifically, aldosterone increases the retention of sodium and the excretion of potassium by the body.

Table 5.1 Social Readjustment Rating Scale

Rank	Life Event	Mean Value
1	Death of spouse	100
2	Divorce	73
3	Marital separation	65
4	Jail term	63
5	Death of a close family member	63
6	Personal injury or illness	53
7	Marriage	50
8	Fired at work	47
9	Marital reconciliation	45
10	Retirement	45
11	Change in health of family member	44
12	Pregnancy	40
13	Sex difficulties	39
14	Gain of a new family member	39
15	Business adjustment	39
16	Change in financial state	38
17	Death of a close friend	37
18	Change to different line of work	36
19	Change in number of arguments with spouse	35
20	Large mortgage	31
21	Foreclosure of mortgage or loan	30
22	Change in responsibilities at work	29
23	Son or daughter leaving home	29
24	Trouble with in-laws	29
25	Outstanding personal achievement	28
26	Wife begins or stops work	26
27	Begin or end school	26
28	Change in living conditions	25
29	Revision of personal habits	24
30	Trouble with boss	23
31	Change in work hours or conditions	20
32	Change in residence	20
33	Change in schools	20
34	Change in recreation	19
35	Change in church activities	19
36	Change in social activities	18
37	Small mortgage	17
38	Change in sleeping habits	16
39	Change in number of family get-togethers	15
40	Change in eating habits	15
41	Vacation	13
42	Christmas	12
43	Minor violations of the law	11

The 17-ketosteroids (sex hormones) are also secreted by the adrenals. The primary sex hormone produced by the adrenal is dehydroepiandrosterone (DHEA).

Assessing Adrenal Function

When I suspect that stress is a major factor, I will often perform a study called the *adrenal stress index*. This test measures the level of the adrenal hormones cortisol and DHEA in the saliva. Two laboratories that I use for this test are Diagnos-Techs (1-800-878-3787) and National BioTech Laboratory (1-800-846-6285). Typically what is found in women with PMS, as well as depressed individuals, is an elevated morning cortisol level and a decreased DHEA level. This pattern represents a maladaptive response to stress.

The effects of increased cortisol levels can be depression, mania, nervousness, insomnia, and schizophrenia. Elevated cortisol levels are also well-recognized feature of depression.[2]

Another test that can be used to determine if adrenal dysfunction is contributing to PMS is the *CRH stimulation test.* This test involves administrating an intravenous dosage of corticotropin-releasing hormone and measuring the response in cortisol levels. Women with PMS often have an increased response to CRH.[3] This abnormality usually signifies reduced inhibition by endorphins. In other words, the reduced levels of endorphins typically found in women with PMS result in an increased sensitivity of the adrenal glands to CRH, causing elevated rises in serum cortisol.

The Problem with Too Much Cortisol

Elevated cortisol levels lead to other problems, including impaired glucose (blood sugar) metabolism and depression. One of the key effects of cortisol in causing depression is related to activating an enzyme known as tryptophan oxy-genase.[4] When activated, this enzyme results in less trypto-phan being delivered to the brain. Since the level of serotonin in the brain is dependent upon how much trypto-phan is delivered to the brain, elevated cortisol levels dra-matically reduce the level of serotonin and melatonin in the brain. This mechanism may be one of the key reasons why serotonin levels are so low in women with PMS (this is dis-cussed more fully in Chapter 6).

In addition to reducing serotonin levels, cortisol also regulates serotonin receptors in the brain, making them less sensitive to the serotonin that is available. Addressing elevated cortisol levels is a major factor in the successful treatment of PMS, especially if depression is a major symptom.

Reducing Stress

Here is what I recommend to reduce the negative effects of stress in women with PMS:

1. Develop a regular exercise program.

2. Perform a relaxation technique such as meditation, prayer, biofeedback, and self-hypnosis for at least 10 minutes twice daily. Such relaxation techniques are vital components of a stress management program.

3. Develop positive coping strategies.

4. Follow the dietary guidelines given in Chapter 7. In particular, consume a diet rich in potassium and low in sodium. This dietary recommendation can be achieved easily by increasing the amounts of whole grains, legumes, vegetables, and fruits that you eat while reducing the amount of salt and prepared foods that you consume.

5. Take a high potency multiple vitamin and mineral formula according to the guidelines given in Chapter 8.

Exercise and PMS

Several studies have shown that women engaged in a regular exercise program do not suffer from PMS nearly as often as sedentary women.[5-7] In one of the more thorough studies, mood and physical symptoms during the menstrual cycle were assessed in 97 women who exercised regularly and in a second group of 159 female non-exercisers.[5] Mood scores and physical symptoms assessed throughout the menstrual cycle revealed that exercise has significant effects on negative mood states and physical symptoms. The regular exercisers obtained significantly lower scores on impaired concentration, negative mood, behavior change, and pain.

In another study, 143 women were monitored for five days in each of the three phases of the cycle (mid-cycle, premenstrual, and menstrual).[5] The women were 35 competitive athletes, two groups of exercisers (33 high exercisers and 36 low exercisers), and 39 sedentary women. The high exercisers experienced the greatest positive mood scores and the sedentary women the least. The high exercisers also reported the least depression and anxiety. The differences were most apparent during the premenstrual and menstrual phases. These results are consistent with the belief that women who exercise frequently (but not competitive athletes) are protected from PMS symptoms. (Note: Competitive female athletes tend to suffer from menstrual irregularities, including absence of menstruation [amenorrhea], as a result of low body fat percentage and the stress of extreme exercise.) One of the key benefits provided by regular exercise is protection against the mood deterioration (primarily depression and irritability) of PMS.

These studies provide evidence that women with PMS need to exercise. One of the ways exercise may be positively impacting PMS is through elevations in endorphin levels (discussed below) and lowering of cortisol levels.

Exercise and Mood

Regular exercise may be the most powerful natural antidepressant available. Numerous community and clinical studies have clearly indicated that exercise has profound antidepressant effects. Increased participation in exercise, sports, and physical activities is strongly associated with decreased symptoms of anxiety (restlessness, tension, etc.), depression (feelings that life is not worthwhile, low spirits, etc.), and malaise (rundown feeling, insomnia, etc.). Furthermore, people who participate in regular exercise have higher self-esteem, feel better, and are much happier compared to people who do not exercise.

In at least 100 clinical studies, an exercise program has been used in the treatment of depression. In these studies, physical fitness training was shown to relieve depression and improve self-esteem and work behavior.[8-13] It was further concluded that exercise can be as effective as other antidepressants, including drugs and psychotherapy.

The best exercises are either strength training (weight lifting) or aerobic activities such as walking briskly, jogging, bicycling, cross-country skiing, swimming, aerobic dance, and racquet sports. Performing these activities for at least 30 minutes a day, four times weekly is a worthwhile goal.

Much of the mood-elevating effects of exercise may be attributed to the fact that regular exercise has been shown to increase the body's level of endorphins.[13] When endorphin levels are low, depression occurs. Conversely, when endorphins levels are elevated, so is one's mood. In an interesting study that examined the role of exercise and endorphins in depression, Dennis Lobstein, Ph.D., a professor of exercise psychobiology at the University of New Mexico, compared the beta-endorphin levels and depression profiles of ten joggers versus ten sedentary men of the same age. The ten sedentary men tested out more depressed, perceived greater stress in their lives, and had more stress-circulating hormones and lower levels of beta-endorphins. As Dr. Lobstein stated, this "reaffirms that depression is very sensitive to exercise and helps firm up a biochemical link between physical activity and depression."[14]

Relaxation Exercises to Reduce Stress

Regularly achieving a relaxed state (i.e., learning to calm the mind and body) is extremely important in relieving stress. The *relaxation response* was a term coined by Harvard professor and cardiologist Herbert Benson, M.D,. in the early 1970s to describe a physiological response that is just the opposite of the stress response. With the stress response, the sympathetic nervous system dominates. With the relaxation response, the parasympathetic nervous system dominates.

To achieve the relaxation response, a variety of techniques can be used. It really doesn't matter which technique you choose, in the end they all should produce the same physiological state—a state of deep relaxation. Some of the techniques you can choose from include meditation, prayer, progressive relaxation, self-hypnosis, and biofeedback. The type of relaxation technique best for each person is totally individual. The important thing is that at least 5 to 10 minutes be set aside each day for the performance of a relaxation technique.

Coping Style and PMS

Whether you are aware of it or not, you have a pattern for coping with stress. Unfortunately, most women with PMS tend to employ *negative* coping styles.[15] I term them *negative* because they ultimately do not support good health. If you are to be truly successful in coping with stress, negative coping patterns must be identified and replaced with positive ways of coping. Try to identify below any negative or destructive coping patterns you may have developed in reaction to stress:

Feelings of helplessness

Overeating

Too much television

Emotional outbursts

Overspending

Obsessive or compulsive behavior

Dependence on chemicals

    Drugs, legal and illicit

    Alcohol

    Smoking

Ten Tips to Improve Coping Strategies

1. Don't starve your emotional life. Foster meaningful relationships. Provide time to give and receive love in your life.

2. Learn to be a good listener. Allow the people in your life to really share their feelings and thoughts uninterrupted. Empathize with them; put yourself in their shoes.

3. Don't try to talk over somebody. If you find yourself being interrupted, relax; don't try and out-talk the other person. If you are courteous and allow

them to speak, eventually (unless they are extremely rude) they will respond likewise. If they don't, point out to them that they are interrupting the communication process. You can only do this if you have been a good listener.

4. Avoid aggressive or passive behavior. Be assertive, but express your thoughts and feelings in a kind way to help improve relationships at work and at home.

5. Avoid excessive stress in your life as best you can by avoiding excessive work hours, poor nutrition, and inadequate rest. Get as much sleep as you can.

6. Avoid stimulants such as caffeine and nicotine. Stimulants promote the fight-or-flight response and tend to make people more irritable.

7. Take time to build long-term health and success by performing stress-reduction techniques and deep breathing exercises.

8. Accept gracefully those things over which you have no control. Save your energy for things that you can do something about.

9. Accept yourself. Remember that you are human and will make mistakes along the way. Consider your mistakes to be learning tools.

10. Be patient and tolerant of other people. Follow the Golden Rule.

Final Comments

Various methods of psychotherapy have been used successfully in improving the psychological aspects of PMS. In particular, psychotherapy in the form of biofeedback or short-term individual counseling (especially cognitive therapy, which is further discussed in Chapter 6) have documented clinical efficacy.[16,17] One of the advantages that cognitive therapy has over antidepressant drug therapy in the treatment of PMS is that learning techniques such as cognitive-behavioral coping skills can produce excellent results that will be maintained over time.

6

Depression, Low Levels of Serotonin, and PMS

There are some important relationships between PMS and depression. Depression is a common feature in many cases of PMS and PMS symptoms are typically more severe in depressed women.[1] The reason appears to be a decrease in the brain level of various neurotransmitters, with serotonin and gamma-aminobutyric acid (GABA) being the most significant.[2,3] Anti-depressant drugs such as Prozac are quickly becoming the dominant medical treatment for PMS.[1] As stated earlier in this book, 80% of the 12 million Americans on Prozac are women between the ages of 25 and 50, also the population with the highest frequency of PMS.

Are You Depressed?

A widely used test for determining depression is the CES-D (Center for Epidemiological Studies–Depression) test developed by Lenore Radloff at the National Institute for Mental Health. This self-test does not diagnose clinical depression, but it can be used to determine your relative level of depression. Simply circle the best description of how you have felt over the past week in the questionnaire on page 49.

To score your test, simply add up all the numbers that you circled. If your score was from 0 to 9, congratulations!, depression is probably not a problem for you. If your score was 10 to 15, you may be mildly depressed. A score between 16 and 24 indicates that depression may be more of a problem for you. If your score was over 24, you are most likely very depressed.

The Biogenic Amine Hypothesis of Depression and PMS

The dominant theoretical model of depression is the *biogenic amine* hypothesis. This model focuses on biochemical factors in the brain causing depression. According to the biogenic amine hypothesis, depression (as well as PMS) is due to a biochemical deficiency characterized by imbalances of amino acids, which form neurotransmitters known as *monoamines.* Monoamines include serotonin, GABA, melatonin, dopamine, and norepinephrine. Environmental, nutritional, hormonal, psychological, and genetic factors can all lead to an imbalance in the monoamines that might result in depression.

A monoamine neurotransmitter is released by brain cells in order to carry a chemical message by binding to receptor sites on neighboring brain cells. Almost as soon as the monoamine is released, enzymes are at work that will either break down the monoamine or work to uptake the monoamine back into the brain cell. Antidepressant drugs act by increasing the level of monoamines in the brain by blocking the re-uptake (e.g., serotonin re-uptake

Depression Test

1. I was bothered by things that usually don't bother me.
   0 Rarely or none of the time (less than 1 day)
   1 Some or a little of the time (1–2 days)
   2 Occasionally or a moderate amount of the time (3–4 days)
   3 Most or all of the time (5–7 days)
2. I did not feel like eating; my appetite was poor.
   0 Rarely or none of the time (less than 1 day)
   1 Some or a little of the time (1–2 days)
   2 Occasionally or a moderate amount of the time (3–4 days)
   3 Most or all of the time (5–7 days)
3. I felt that I could not shake off the blues even with help from my family and friends.
   0 Rarely or none of the time (less than 1 day)
   1 Some or a little of the time (1–2 days)
   2 Occasionally or a moderate amount of the time (3–4 days)
   3 Most or all of the time (5–7 days)
4. I felt that I was not as good as other people.
   0 Rarely or none of the time (less than 1 day)
   1 Some or a little of the time (1–2 days)
   2 Occasionally or a moderate amount of the time (3–4 days)
   3 Most or all of the time (5–7 days)
5. I had trouble keeping my mind on what I was doing.
   0 Rarely or none of the time (less than 1 day)
   1 Some or a little of the time (1–2 days)
   2 Occasionally or a moderate amount of the time (3–4 days)
   3 Most or all of the time (5–7 days)
6. I felt depressed.
   0 Rarely or none of the time (less than 1 day)
   1 Some or a little of the time (1–2 days)
   2 Occasionally or a moderate amount of the time (3–4 days)
   3 Most or all of the time (5–7 days)
7. I felt like everything I did was an effort.
   0 Rarely or none of the time (less than 1 day)
   1 Some or a little of the time (1–2 days)
   2 Occasionally or a moderate amount of the time (3–4 days)
   3 Most or all of the time (5–7 days)
8. I felt hopeless about the future.
   0 Rarely or none of the time (less than 1 day)
   1 Some or a little of the time (1–2 days)
   2 Occasionally or a moderate amount of the time (3–4 days)
   3 Most or all of the time (5–7 days)

Depression Test (continued)

9. I thought my life had been a failure.

   0   Rarely or none of the time (less than 1 day)
   1   Some or a little of the time (1–2 days)
   2   Occasionally or a moderate amount of the time (3–4 days)
   3   Most or all of the time (5–7 days)

10. I felt fearful.

   0   Rarely or none of the time (less than 1 day)
   1   Some or a little of the time (1–2 days)
   2   Occasionally or a moderate amount of the time (3–4 days)
   3   Most or all of the time (5–7 days)

11. My sleep was restless.

   0   Rarely or none of the time (less than 1 day)
   1   Some or a little of the time (1–2 days)
   2   Occasionally or a moderate amount of the time (3–4 days)
   3   Most or all of the time (5–7 days)

12. I was unhappy.

   0   Rarely or none of the time (less than 1 day)
   1   Some or a little of the time (1–2 days)
   2   Occasionally or a moderate amount of the time (3–4 days)
   3   Most or all of the time (5–7 days)

13. I talked less than usual.

   0   Rarely or none of the time (less than 1 day)
   1   Some or a little of the time (1–2 days)
   2   Occasionally or a moderate amount of the time (3–4 days)
   3   Most or all of the time (5–7 days)

14. I felt lonely.

   0   Rarely or none of the time (less than 1 day)
   1   Some or a little of the time (1–2 days)
   2   Occasionally or a moderate amount of the time (3–4 days)
   3   Most or all of the time (5–7 days)

15. People were unfriendly.

   0   Rarely or none of the time (less than 1 day)
   1   Some or a little of the time (1–2 days)
   2   Occasionally or a moderate amount of the time (3–4 days)
   3   Most or all of the time (5–7 days)

16. I did not enjoy life.

   0   Rarely or none of the time (less than 1 day)
   1   Some or a little of the time (1–2 days)
   2   Occasionally or a moderate amount of the time (3–4 days)
   3   Most or all of the time (5–7 days)

Depression Test *(continued)*

17. I had crying spells.
    - 0 Rarely or none of the time (less than 1 day)
    - 1 Some or a little of the time (1–2 days)
    - 2 Occasionally or a moderate amount of the time (3–4 days)
    - 3 Most or all of the time (5–7 days)

18. I felt sad.
    - 0 Rarely or none of the time (less than 1 day)
    - 1 Some or a little of the time (1–2 days)
    - 2 Occasionally or a moderate amount of the time (3–4 days)
    - 3 Most or all of the time (5–7 days)

19. I felt that people disliked me.
    - 0 Rarely or none of the time (less than 1 day)
    - 1 Some or a little of the time (1–2 days)
    - 2 Occasionally or a moderate amount of the time (3–4 days)
    - 3 Most or all of the time (5–7 days)

20. I could not get "going."
    - 0 Rarely or none of the time (less than 1 day)
    - 1 Some or a little of the time (1–2 days)
    - 2 Occasionally or a moderate amount of the time (3–4 days)
    - 3 Most or all of the time (5–7 days)

Total Score: _____

inhibitors), blocking the breakdown (by inhibiting the enzyme monoamine oxidase), or enhancing the effect of a specific monoamine (e.g., the tricyclic antidepressant drugs).

Serotonin Re-Uptake Inhibitors and PMS

Prozac and several other drugs (e.g., Effexor, Paxil, and Zoloft) classified as *serotonin re-uptake inhibitors* (SRIs) are becoming the first line of therapy in the treatment of PMS by the conventional medical establishment.[1] These drugs inhibit the re-uptake of serotonin at the nerve endings in the brain. As a result, more serotonin is likely to bind to receptor sites on brain cells and transmit the serotonin signal. Serotonin, a very important neurotransmitter, is the brain's own natural antidepressant and tranquilizer. A decrease in serotonin function is thought to be a major cause of depression, anxiety, insomnia, carbohydrate craving, and PMS. Fortunately, natural alternatives to Prozac and other antidepressant drugs are as effective without the risk of side effects. Chief among these natural alternatives is St. John's wort extract.

St. John's Wort Extract

Over 25 double-blind, controlled trials (15 versus placebo, 10 versus standard anti-depressant drugs) have shown that St. John's wort (*Hypericum perforatum*) extracts standardized for hypericin yield excellent results in the treatment of depression with virtually no side effects. Yet most American physicians have even never heard of St. John's wort extract.

In contrast, it is estimated that nearly 70% of all German physicians regularly prescribe botanical medicines. The fastest rising star in botanical medicine in Germany is St. John's wort. The total of 66 million daily doses of St. John's wort preparations prescribed by German physicians in 1994 are expected to be dramatically higher when tallied for 1995, 1996, and beyond.

The obvious questions is: Why do so many German M.D.s know about St. John's wort, Ginkgo, and other herbal medicines while American M.D.s remain ignorant? In an editorial in the January 1995 issue of *The American Journal of Natural Medicine,* Mark Blumenthal, Executive Director of the American Botanical Council, described the system in Germany that helps physicians make informed choices regarding botanical medicines. German authorities have developed a series of monographs (now totaling over 400) developed by Commission E, an independent division of the German Federal Health Agency, which describe the clinical uses of herbal preparations. Commission E evaluates efficacy of herbal medicines based on a doctrine of reasonable certainty versus the U.S. FDA's doctrine of absolute proof. Herbal products can be marketed with drug claims if they have been proven to be safe and effective. Whether the herbal product is available by prescription or over the counter is based upon its application and safety of use. Herbal products sold in pharmacies are reimbursed by insurance if they are prescribed by a physician.

Because the German system allows companies to market their products according to the guidelines of Commission E, many companies achieved success with their products. They were then able to fund the necessary research to gain greater acceptance within mainstream conventional medicine. The case of St. John's wort extract in the treatment of depression is a perfect illustration of how the Commission E monographs have led to significant documentation of a plant with a long history of folk use for depression.

If you would like more information on Germany's Commission E or the efforts going on in the United States regarding the adoption of similar guidelines, contact the American Botanical Council. This nonprofit organization dedicated to advancing botanical medicine in the United States is the publisher of *HerbalGram* and has recently translated Commission E monographs into English. For more information, contact:

The American Botanical Council
P.O. Box 201660
Austin, TX 78720-1660
(512) 331-8868
(512) 331-1924 fax

How Does St. John's Wort Work?

When the Commission E monograph for St. John's wort came out in 1984 it identified the constituent hypericin as an experimental monoamine oxidase inhibitor and permitted the medicinal use of the herb in average doses of 2 to 4 g of herb, or 0.2 to 1.0 mg total hypericin, for depression, anxiety, or nervous excitement.

Because of this relative endorsement by Commission E, companies were able to fund research to better understand the way in which St. John's wort appeared to be effective for these disorders. The results from this research are fueling the tremendous popularity of St. John's wort extract in Germany and its growing popularity in the United States.

Originally it was thought that hypericin acted as an inhibitor of the enzyme monoamine oxidase—thereby resulting in the increase of brain monoamines such as serotonin and dopamine. However, newer information indicates that St. John's wort possesses no in vivo inhibition of monoamine oxidase.[4] It appears that the antidepressant activities are more related to modulating the relationship between the immune system and mood as well as inhibiting serotonin re-uptake in a way similar to the SRI drugs such as Prozac, Paxil, and Zoloft.[5,6] In addition, it appears that while hypericin is an important marker, other compounds, such as flavonoids, are thought to play a major role in the pharmacology of St. John's wort.

Results from Clinical Studies

Although the exact mechanism of action for the antidepressant effects of St. John's wort extract has not yet been fully determined, based on the results of the double-blind clinical trials, it is an effective antidepressant in cases of mild to moderately severe depression.

A recent meta-analysis of all of the studies featuring the use of St. John's wort for depression appeared in the *British Medical Journal*.[7] A *meta-analysis* refers to analysis of the combined results from a number of selected trials in order to arrive at a general conclusion. In this meta-analysis, 23 double-blind randomized trials involving a total of 1,757 outpatients with mild to moderately severe depression were analyzed. The results indicated that St. John's wort extracts were significantly superior to placebo and as effective as standard antidepressant drugs.

St. John's Wort Versus Prozac

If St. John's wort was only as effective as standard antidepressant drugs, why use it? Safety. While standard antidepressant drugs are successful in alleviating depression in many cases (60% to 75%), they are also associated with many side effects. Prozac is generally regarded as being better tolerated largely based on the fact that only 17% of patients taking Prozac discontinue treatment because of side effects compared to 31% of patients taking a tricyclic antidepressant. However, Prozac is regarded as being "better tolerated" only because side effects are so common with the other antidepressant drugs. Prozac is far from being classified as a well-tolerated drug. Results from clinical trials have demonstrated that 21% of patients taking the drug experience nausea, 20% headaches, 15% anxiety and nervousness, 14% insomnia, 12% drowsiness, 12% diarrhea, 9.5% dry mouth, 9% loss of appetite, 8% sweating and tremor, and 3% rash.[8] Prozac and other antidepressants inhibit sexual function. In studies where sexual side effects were thoroughly evaluated, 43% of men and women taking various antidepressants and 34% taking Prozac reported loss of libido or diminished sexual response.[9] Surprisingly, the latest edition of the *Physician's Desk Reference* lists that only 2% of patients suffer from sexual problems as a result of Prozac. This discrepancy is substantial and probably reflects the difficulty in feeling comfortable talking about a sensitive subject by patients. Thus, the 43% level is probably more reflective of the degree of sexual problems caused by Prozac.

Prozac is more likely than other antidepressants to cause a condition called *akathisia*—a drug-induced state of agitation. In some people, it may induce violent and destructive outbursts. The violent and suicidal reactions experienced by some patients taking Prozac have become so common and publicized that several citizens groups have formed to create awareness of the dangers of this drug. Although several studies have not shown an association between Prozac and suicide, these studies are offset by numerous case reports suggesting a strong link between Prozac and suicide.

The Safety of St. John's Wort

In contrast to standard antidepressants, St. John's wort extract is virtually free of side effects at the standard dosage. The frequency and severity of side effects with St. John's wort extract are clinically insignificant, especially when compared to the well-known side effects of Prozac and other antidepressants.

The standard dosage of St. John's wort extract (0.3% hypericin) is 300 mg three times daily. No significant side effects have been reported in the numerous double-blind studies, but perhaps the best demonstration of the excellent safety record of St. John's wort extract is a large scale study involving 3,250 patients, which was conducted in Germany.[10] Results were analyzed by means of a patient questionnaire. Pooled data indicated that symptoms of depression were reduced in frequency and intensity by approximately 50%. The undesired side effects were reported in 79 patients (2.43%) and 48 (1.45%) discontinued therapy. The most frequently noted side effects were gastrointestinal irritation (0.55%), allergic reactions (0.52%), fatigue (0.4%), and restlessness (0.26%).

The scientific investigation of St. John's wort is certainly not complete. There is still much to be learned and demonstrated. From a clinical perspective, the major shortcomings of the existing clinical trials is their relatively short term (8 weeks) and the lack of studies of severely depressed patients. Given its growing popularity, studies that address these shortcoming are surely forthcoming. What can be concluded from currently available information is that St. John's wort extract is quite appropriate as an alternative to standard antidepressant drugs in cases of mild to moderate depression. Whether it will be shown to be suitable in the treatment of serious depression (i.e., depression associated with psychotic symptoms and/or depression with serious risk of suicide) remains to be answered. Fortunately, mild to moderately severe depression is far more common than severe depression.

Dealing with Depression Naturally

In my book *Natural Alternatives to Prozac* (Morrow, 1996) I thoroughly discussed natural alternatives to anti-depressant drugs such as Prozac. Rather than relying on drugs to alter brain chemistry, the natural approach provides the brain with the support it needs to function optimally. If depression is a major factor in your life, I want to encourage you to get my book and follow the recommendations given. In the meantime, here are ten recommendations to follow:

1. Develop a positive, optimistic mental attitude by:
   Setting goals
   Using positive affirmations
   Asking yourself empowering questions
   Seeking the help of a mental health professional
2. If you smoke, get help to quit
3. Avoid the intake of caffeine or other stimulants and alcohol
4. Exercise regularly
5. Perform a relaxation/stress-reduction technique for 10 to 15 minutes each day
6. Find ways to interject humor and laughter in your life
7. Eat a healthful diet as outlined in Chapter 7
8. Take a high-potency multiple vitamin and mineral formula as outlined in Chapter 8
9. Take one tablespoon of flaxseed oil daily to obtain the essential fatty acids that your body needs (see Chapter 8)
10. Take St. John's wort extract (0.3% hypericin content) at a dosage of 300 mg, three times daily

Final Comments

If you suffer PMS with severe irritability or depression, I also strongly encourage you to consult a psychotherapist; there are a number of psychological therapies that can be quite useful in helping to eliminate depression. The therapy that has the most support in the medical literature is called *cognitive therapy.* In fact, cognitive therapy has been shown to be equally as effective as antidepressant drugs in treating moderate depression.[11,12] However, while there is a high rate of relapse of depression when drugs are used, the relapse rate for cognitive therapy is much lower. People taking drugs for depression often have to stay on them for the rest of their lives. That is not the case with cognitive therapy because the patient is taught new skills to deal with depression.[13]

Psychologists and other mental health specialists trained in cognitive therapy seek to change the way depressed persons consciously think about failure, defeat, loss, and helplessness. Cognitive therapists employ five basic tactics.

First they help patients to recognize the negative thoughts that flit automatically through their consciousness at the times when they feel the worst. The second tactic is disputing the negative thoughts by focusing on contrary evidence. The third tactic is teaching the patients a different explanation to dispute the negative automatic thoughts. The fourth tactic involves learning how to avoid rumination (the constant churning of a thought in one's mind) by helping the patients better control their thoughts. The final tactic is questioning depression-causing negative thoughts and beliefs, and replacing them with empowering positive thoughts and beliefs.

Cognitive therapy does not involve the long, drawn-out process of psychoanalysis. It is a solution-oriented psychotherapy designed to help patients learn skills that can improve the quality of their lives. If your thought processes are in need of a little rewiring, please consult a mental health specialist that practices cognitive therapy.

7

Dietary Guidelines

Successful treatment of PMS usually involves making some dietary changes. Most women in the United States eat the so-called *SAD* (*Standard American Diet*). This diet does not promote health nor does it support proper estrogen metabolism. As a result, female complaints such as PMS, fibrocystic breast disease, uterine fibroids, and, more seriously, breast cancer are much more frequent in American women compared to women in many other parts of the world. Women suffering from PMS typically eat a diet that is even worse than the SAD. Guy Abraham, M.D. reports that, compared to symptom-free women, PMS patients consume 62% more refined carbohydrates, 275% more refined sugar, 79% more dairy products, 78% more sodium, 53% less iron, 77% less manganese, and 52% less zinc.[1]

In addition to providing benefits against PMS symptoms, the dietary recommendations provided in this chapter provide significant protection against the development of breast cancer, other cancers, heart disease, strokes, osteoporosis, diabetes, and virtually every other chronic degenerative disease.

The seven most important dietary recommendations for PMS are:

1. Follow a vegetarian or predominantly vegetarian diet.
2. Reduce your intake of fat.
3. Eliminate sugar.
4. Reduce your exposure to environmental estrogens.
5. Increase your intake of soy foods.
6. Eliminate caffeine.
7. Keep your salt intake low.

Following a Vegetarian Diet

Vegetarian women have been shown to excrete two to three times more estrogen in their feces and have 50% lower levels of free estrogen in their blood compared to omnivores.[2,3] These differences are thought to be a result of the lower fat and higher fiber intake of the vegetarian women. These dietary differences also may explain the lower incidence of breast cancer, heart disease, and menopausal symptoms in vegetarian women.

At the very least, eat less saturated fat and cholesterol by reducing or eliminating the amounts of animal products in your diet and increase your consumption of fiber-rich plant foods (fruits, vegetables, grains, and legumes). Limit your intake of animal protein sources to no more than 4 to 6 ounces per day and choose fish, skinless poultry, and lean cuts rather than fat-laden choices.

Be sure to eat five or more servings of a combination of vegetables and fruits, especially green and yellow vegetables and citrus fruits, each day. Many medical experts

Table 7.1   Food Choices for Lowering Cholesterol and
Estrogen Levels

Eat Less of These	Substitute with These
Red meats	Fish and white meat of poultry
Hamburgers and hot dogs	Soy-based alternatives
Eggs	Egg Beaters and similar products, tofu
High-fat dairy products	Lowfat or nonfat dairy products, soy milk
Butter, lard, and other saturated fats	Vegetable oils
Ice cream, pies, cake, cookies, etc.	Fruits
Refined cereals, white bread, etc.	Whole grains, whole wheat bread
Fried foods, fatty snack foods	Vegetables, fresh salads
Salt and salty foods	Low sodium foods, light salt
Coffee and soft drinks	Herbal teas, fresh fruit and vegetable juices

and departments of the U.S. government including the U.S. National Academy of Science, the U.S. Department of Agriculture, the U.S. Department of Health and Human Services, the National Research Council, and the National Cancer Institute recommend that Americans consume two to three serving of fruit and three to five servings of vegetables per day to reduce the risk of developing heart disease, cancer, and other chronic degenerative diseases. Unfortunately, less than 10% of the population are meeting even the lowest recommendation of five servings of a combination of fruits and vegetables per day.

Numerous population studies have repeatedly demonstrated that a high intake of carotene- and flavonoid-rich fruits and vegetables reduces the risk of cancer, heart disease, and strokes.[4,5] Carotenes represent the most widespread group of naturally occurring pigments in nature. They are a highly colored (red and yellow) group of fat-soluble compounds. Over 600 carotenoids have been identified, including 30 to 50 that the body can transform into vitamin A. Beta-carotene has been termed the most active of the carotenoids, due to its higher provitamin A activity, but several other carotenes exert greater antioxidant effects.

The best dietary sources of carotenes are green leafy vegetables and yellow- or orange-colored fruits and vegetables—e.g., carrots, apricots, mangoes, yams, and squash. Red and purple vegetables and fruits—such as tomatoes, red cabbage, berries, and plums—contain a large portion of carotenes and flavonoids. Legumes, grains, and seeds are also significant sources of carotenoids.

The flavonoids are another group of plant pigments that provide remarkable protection against cancer, heart disease, and strokes. These compounds are largely responsible for the colors of fruits and flowers. Flavonoids act as powerful antioxidants in providing protection against oxidative and free radical damage. Good dietary sources of flavonoids include citrus fruits, berries, onions, parsley, legumes, green tea, and red wine. Given the potent antioxidant protection provided by flavonoids, increasing consumption of high-flavonoid sources is an important dietary goal.

Many of the effects that a vegetarian diet has on lowering circulating estrogen levels are related to a higher intake of dietary fiber. The fiber promotes the excretion of estrogens directly and indirectly by promoting a more favorable bacterial flora with lower levels of beta-glucuronidase activity. In an attempt to help my patients increase their intake of high-fiber foods, I will often instruct them to try to achieve total daily intake of 25 to 35 grams of fiber from the foods listed in Table 7.2.

Table 7.2   Dietary Fiber Content of Selected Foods

Food	Serving	Calories	Grams of Fiber
Fruits (no more than 4 servings daily)			
Apple (with skin)	1 medium	81	3.5
Banana	1 medium	105	2.4
Cantaloupe	¼ melon	30	1.0
Cherries, sweet	10	49	1.2
Grapefruit	½ medium	38	1.6
Orange	1 medium	62	2.6
Peach (with skin)	1	37	1.9
Pear (with skin)	½ large	61	3.1
Prunes	3	60	3.0
Raisins	¼ cup	106	3.1
Raspberries	½ cup	35	3.1
Strawberries	1 cup	45	3.0
Vegetables, Raw (as many servings as desired)			
Bean sprouts	½ cup	13	1.5
Celery, diced	½ cup	10	1.1
Cucumber	½ cup	8	0.4
Lettuce	1 cup	10	0.9
Mushrooms	½ cup	10	1.5
Pepper, green	½ cup	9	0.5
Spinach	1 cup	8	1.2
Tomato	1 medium	20	1.5
Vegetables, Cooked			
Asparagus, cut	1 cup	30	2.0
Beans, green	1 cup	32	3.2
Broccoli	1 cup	40	4.4
Brussels sprouts	1 cup	56	4.6
Cabbage	1 cup	30	2.8
Carrots	1 cup	48	4.6
Cauliflower	1 cup	28	2.2
Corn	½ cup	87	2.9
Kale	1 cup	44	2.8
Parsnip	1 cup	102	5.4
Potato (with skin)	1 medium	106	2.5
Potato (without skin)	1 medium	97	1.4
Spinach	1 cup	42	4.2
Sweet potato	1 medium	160	3.4
Zucchini	1 cup	22	3.6

Table 7.2 Dietary Fiber Content of Selected Foods *(continued)*

Food	Serving	Calories	Grams of Fiber
Legumes			
Baked beans	½ cup	155	8.8
Dried peas, cooked	½ cup	115	4.7
Kidney beans, cooked	½ cup	110	7.3
Lima beans, cooked	½ cup	164	4.5
Lentils, cooked	½ cup	97	3.7
Navy beans, cooked	½ cup	112	6.0
Breakfast Cereals (no more than 2 servings daily)			
All-Bran	⅓ cup	71	8.5
Bran Chex	⅔ cup	91	4.6
Corn Bran	⅔ cup	98	5.4
Oatmeal	¾ cup	108	1.6
Raisin Bran	⅔ cup	115	4.0
Shredded Wheat	⅔ cup	102	2.6

Reducing Your Intake of Fat

Decreasing the percentage of calories consumed as fat, in particular saturated fat, has dramatic effects on reducing circulating estrogen.[6,7] In one study, when 17 women switched from the SAD (40% of calories as fat and only 12 grams of fiber) to a lowfat, high-fiber diet (25% of calories as fat and 40 grams of fiber) there was a 36% reduction in blood estrogen levels, with 16 out of the 17 women demonstrating significant reductions in only 8 to 10 weeks.[6] A lowfat diet has also been shown to improve PMS symptoms.[8]

Another good reason to reduce your intake of fat is the great deal of research linking a diet high in saturated fat and cholesterol to numerous cancers, heart disease, and strokes. Both the American Cancer Society and the American Heart Association recommend a diet containing less than 30% of calories as fat.

Looking at Table 7.3 it is obvious that the easiest way for most people to achieve this goal is to eat less animal products and more plant foods. With the exception of nuts and seeds, most plant foods are very low in fat. In regard to nuts and seeds, the calories are derived largely from polyunsaturated essential fatty acids, which are much more healthful than saturated fats.

It is also very important to eliminate your intake of margarine and foods containing trans-fatty acids and partially-hydrogenated oils. During the process of margarine and shortening manufacture, vegetable oils are *hydrogenated.* This means that a hydrogen molecule is added to the natural unsaturated fatty acid molecules of the vegetable oil to make them more saturated (solid). Hydrogenation results in changing the structure of the natural fatty acid to many "unnatural" fatty acid forms, which interfere with the body's ability to utilize essential fatty acids.

Many researchers and nutritionists have been concerned about the health effects of margarine since it was first introduced. Although many Americans assume that they are doing their body good by consuming margarine instead butter (a saturated fat), in truth they are actually doing more harm. Margarine and other hydrogenated vegetable oils not only raise LDL cholesterol, they also lower the protective HDL cholesterol level, interfere with essential fatty acid metabolism, and are suspected of being causes of certain cancers (including breast cancer).[9]

Eliminating Sugar

Sugar has several detrimental actions in PMS. First of all, when high-sugar foods are eaten alone, blood-sugar levels rise quickly, producing a strain on blood-sugar control. Eating foods high in simple sugars can be harmful to blood-sugar control—especially if you are hypoglycemic or

Table 7.3 Fat Content (as a Percentage of Calories) of Selected Foods

Meats		Vegetables	
Sirloin steak, hipbone, lean w/fat	83%	Mustard greens	13%
Pork sausage	83%	Kale	13%
T-bone steak, lean w/fat	82%	Beet greens	12%
Porterhouse steak, lean w/fat	82%	Lettuce	12%
Bacon, lean	82%	Turnip greens	11%
Rib roast, lean w/fat	81%	Mushrooms	8%
Bologna	81%	Cabbage	7%
Country-style sausage	81%	Cauliflower	7%
Spareribs	80%	Eggplant	7%
Frankfurters	80%	Asparagus	6%
Lamb rib chops, lean w/fat	79%	Green beens	6%
Duck meat, w/skin	76%	Celery	6%
Salami	76%	Cucumber	6%
Liverwurst	75%	Turnip	6%
Rump roast, lean w/fat	71%	Zucchini	6%
Ham, lean w/fat	69%	Carrots	4%
Stewing beef, lean w/fat	66%	Green peas	4%
Goose meat, w/skin	65%	Artichokes	3%
Ground beef, fairly lean	64%	Onions	3%
Veal breast, lean w/fat	64%	Beets	2%
Leg of lamb, lean w/fat	61%	Chives	1%
Chicken, dark meat w/skin, roasted	56%	Potatoes	1%
Round steak, lean w/fat	53%	*Legumes*	
Chuck rib roast, lean only	50%	Tofu	49%
Sirloin steak, hipbone, lean only	47%	Soybean	37%
Turkey, dark meat w/skin	47%	Soybean sprouts	28%
Lamb rib chops, lean only	45%	Garbanzo bean	11%
Chicken, light meat w/skin, roasted	44%	Kidney bean	4%
		Lima bean	4%
		Mungbean sprouts	4%
Fish		Lentil	3%
Tuna, chunk, oil-packed	63%	Broad bean	3%
Herring, Pacific	59%	Mung bean	3%
Anchovies	54%		
Bass, black sea	53%		
Perch, ocean	53%		
Caviar, sturgeon	52%		
Mackerel, Pacific	50%		
Sardines, Atlantic, in oil, drained	49%		
Salmon, sockeye (red)	49%		

Table 7.3 Fat Content (as a Percentage of Calories) of Selected Foods

Dairy Products		Fruits	
Butter	100%	Olive	91%
Cream, light whipping	92%	Avocado	82%
Cream cheese	90%	Grape	11%
Cream, light or coffee	85%	Strawberry	11%
Egg yolks	80%	Apple	8%
Half and half	79%	Blueberry	7%
Blue cheese	73%	Lemon	7%
Brick cheese	72%	Pear	5%
Cheddar cheese	71%	Apricot	4%
Swiss cheese	66%	Orange	4%
Ricotta cheese, whole-milk	66%	Cherry	4%
type		Banana	4%
Eggs, whole	65%	Cantaloupe	3%
Mozzarella cheese,	55%	Pineapple	3%
part skim type		Grapefruit	2%
Goat's milk	54%	Papaya	2%
Cow's milk, whole	49%	Peach	2%
Yogurt, plain	49%	Prune	1%
Ice cream, regular	48%	*Grains*	
Cottage cheese	35%	Oatmeal	16%
Lowfat milk (2%)	31%	Buckwheat, dark	7%
Lowfat yogurt (2%)	31%	Rye, dark	7%
Ice milk	29%	Whole wheat	5%
Nonfat cottage cheese (1%)	22%	Brown rice	5%
Meat and Fish Products		Corn flour	5%
Hormel Spam luncheon meat	77%	Bulgur	4%
Mrs. Paul's Buttered	75%	Barley	3%
Fish Fillets		Buckwheat, light	2%
Del Monte Bonito	67%	Wild rice	2%
Morton Beef Tenderloin	64%	*Nuts and Seeds*	
Mrs. Paul's Fried Shrimp	58%	Coconut	85%
Mrs. Paul's Clam Crepes	55%	Walnut	79%
Hormel Dinty Moore	53%	Sesame	76%
Corned Beef		Almond	76%
Swanson Salisbury Steak	52%	Sunflower	71%
Morton House Beef Stew	49%	Pumpkin seeds	71%
Mrs. Paul's Flounder	48%	Cashew	70%
Swanson Veal Parmigiana	48%	Peanut	69%
Swanson Fried Chicken	46%	Chestnut	7%
Hormel Dinty Moore	45%		
Beef Stew			
Morton Beef Pot Pie	45%	*Source: "Nutritive Value of Ameri-*	
Mrs. Paul's Fish Au Gratin	43%	*can Foods in Common Units,"*	
Morton Chicken Croquettes	40%	*U.S.D.A. Handbook No. 456.*	

diabetic. Sugar, especially when combined with caffeine, also has a detrimental effect on PMS and mood (discussed below). The most significant symptom-producing food in PMS appears to be chocolate.[10]

Another detrimental effect of a high intake of sugar is impaired estrogen metabolism.[11] The evidence is based on the higher frequency of PMS symptoms in women consuming a high-sugar diet and the fact that a high-sugar intake is also associated with higher estrogen levels.[1]

Read food labels carefully for clues on sugar content. If the words *sucrose, glucose, maltose, lactose, fructose, corn syrup* or *white grape juice concentrate* appear on the label, extra sugar has been added. Currently, more than half of the carbohydrates being consumed by most Americans are in the form of sugars that have been added to foods as sweetening agents.[6]

Reducing Your Exposure to Environmental Estrogens

Widespread environmental contamination has occurred with a group of compounds known as *halogenated hydrocarbons.* Included in this group are the toxic pesticides DDT, DDE, PCB, PCP, dieldrin, and chlordane. These molecules are hard to break down and, once ingested, are stored in fat cells. These chemicals are known to mimic estrogen in the body and are thought to be a major factor in the growing epidemics of estrogen-related health problems such as PMS, breast cancer, and low sperm counts.[12,13]

Pesticide residue levels in food are monitored by both state and federal regulatory agencies. Such monitoring is used to enforce legal tolerance levels. However, there has been increasing public concern about the adequacy of the residue monitoring programs. While the EPA and FDA estimate that excessive pesticide residues are found on about 3% of domestic and 6% of foreign produce, other organizations report much higher estimates.

For example, the National Resources Defense Council conducted a survey of fresh produce sold in San Francisco markets for pesticide residues and found that 44% of 71 fruits and vegetables had detectable levels of 19 different pesticides; 42% of the produce had detectable pesticide residues containing more than one pesticide.[14]

The sheer number and amount of pesticides showered on certain foods is astounding. For example, over 50 different pesticides are used on broccoli, 110 on apples, 70 on bell peppers, and so on.[15] Because many of the pesticides penetrate the entire fruit or vegetable and cannot be washed off, it is obviously best to buy organic.

Many supermarket chains and produce suppliers employ their own testing measures for determining the pesticide content of produce and are refusing to stock foods that have been treated with some of the more toxic pesticides, such as alachlor, captan, or EBDCs (ethylene bisdithiocarbamates). In addition, many stores are asking growers to disclose all pesticides used on their produce as well as phase out the use of the 64 pesticides suspected of being capable of causing cancers. Ultimately it will be pressure from consumers that will influence food suppliers the most. Crop yield studies support the use of organic farming if the risk to human health is added to the equation.

Avoiding Pesticides

1. Since pesticide residues (even in organically raised animals) are concentrated in animal fat, meat, eggs, cheese, and milk, it makes good sense to avoid these foods.

2. Buy organic produce. In the context of food and farming, the term *organic* is used to imply that the

produce was grown without the aid of synthetic chemicals, including pesticides and fertilizers. In 1973, Oregon became the first state to pass laws that define labeling laws for organic produce. By 1989, 16 other states (California, Colorado, Iowa, Maine, Massachusetts, Minnesota, Montana, Nebraska, New Hampshire, North Dakota, Ohio, South Dakota, Texas, Vermont, Washington, and Wisconsin) had also adopted state laws governing organic agriculture. Consumers should ask if the produce is *certified organic* and if so, by whom. Highly reputable certification organizations include California Certified Organic Farmers, Demeter, Farm Verified Organic, Natural Organic Farmers Association, and the Organic Crop Improvement Association. Although under 3% of the total produce grown in the United States is grown without the aid of pesticides, organic produce is widely available.

3. If organic produce is not readily available in your area, develop a good relationship with your local grocery store produce manager. Explain your desire to reduce your exposure to pesticides and waxes. Ask what measures the store takes to ensure that pesticide residues are within the tolerance limits. Ask where they get their produce; foreign produce is much more likely to contain excessive levels of pesticides as well as pesticides that have been banned in the United States due to suspected toxicity. Try to buy local produce that is in season.

4. To remove surface pesticide residues, waxes, fungicides, and fertilizers, soak the produce in a mild solution of additive-free soap such as Ivory or pure castile soap from the health food store. You can also use an all-natural, biodegradable cleanser available at most health food stores. Simply spray

the produce with the cleaner, gently scrub, and then rinse off. Another technique is to simply peel off the skin or remove the outer layer of leaves. The down side of this is that many of the nutritional benefits are concentrated in the skin and outer layers.

The presence of pesticides in fruits and vegetables should not deter you from eating a diet high in these foods because the concentrations in fruits and vegetables are much lower than the levels found in animal fats, meat, cheese, whole milk, and eggs. Furthermore, the various antioxidant components in fruits and vegetables help the body deal with the pesticides.

Increasing Your Intake of Soy Foods

Soy and soy foods contain compounds referred to as *phytoestrogens* because they are capable of binding to estrogen receptors. Phytoestrogens are also often referred to as *antiestrogens* because their estrogenic effect is only 2% as strong as estrogen at the very most. However, because of this low activity, phytoestrogens have a balancing action on estrogen's effects. If estrogen levels are low (as in menopause), since phytoestrogens have some estrogenic activity, they will cause an increase in estrogen effect. If estrogen levels are high (as in PMS), since phytoestrogens bind to estrogen receptors, thereby competing with estrogen, there will be a decrease in estrogen effects.

In June 1990, the National Cancer Institute held a workshop to examine the relationship of soybean consumption to cancer prevention.[16,17] Soybean consumption is thought to be one of the major reasons for the relatively low rate of breast and colon cancers in Japan and China. Studies in animals have demonstrated that diets composed of as little as 5% soybeans can significantly inhibit chemical-induced cancers. The most important anticancer compounds in relation to breast cancer appear to be the phytoestrogens (isoflavonoids and phytosterols).

The soybean plant (*Glycine max*) is native to China, where it has been cultivated for food for well over 13,000 years. The ancient Chinese considered the soybean their most important crop and a necessity for life. The soybean, thanks largely to the United States, which accounts for over 50% of the world's production, is now the most widely grown and utilized legume. In terms of dollar value, the soybean is the most important U.S. crop, ranking above corn, wheat, and cotton. Unfortunately, in the United States, despite its use in a variety of food products, the soybean is still used primarily for animal feed (protein meal) and for its oils. However, since the 1970s, there has been a marked increase in both the consumption of traditional soy foods such as tofu, tempeh, and miso, and in the development of so-called second-generation soy foods that simulate traditional meat and dairy products. Consumers can now find soy flour, soy milk, soy hot dogs, soy sausage, soy cheese, and soy frozen desserts at their grocery stores.

The increase in soy food consumption is attributed to a number of factors, including economics, health benefits, and environmental concerns. In terms of cost, soybeans provide a great amount of nutrition per acre. In fact, an acre of soybeans can provide nearly 20 times the amount of protein that an acre used for raising beef can. The use of soybeans for human consumption will grow as the world's population continues to grow and its food supply continues to shrink.

Soybeans can be utilized in their whole cooked or sprouted form, either on their own or in recipes. Soybeans can substitute for other beans in soups, stews, casseroles, and other dishes. In addition, there are many other soy foods that can be used including soy alternatives to hamburgers, as well as the second-generation soy foods listed above.

Eliminating Caffeine

Caffeine must be avoided by patients with PMS, especially if anxiety or depression or breast tenderness and fibrocystic breast disease are major symptoms.[18,19] Considerable evidence demonstrates that caffeine consumption is strongly related to the presence and severity of PMS. The effect of caffeine is particularly significant in the psychological symptoms associated with PMS, such as anxiety, irritability, insomnia, and depression. The effect of caffeine on fibrocystic breast disease is discussed on page 134.

The average American consumes 150 to 225 mg of caffeine daily, or roughly the amount of caffeine in one to two cups of coffee. Although most people can handle this amount, some people are more sensitive to the effects of caffeine than others. Even small amounts of caffeine, as found in decaffeinated coffee, are enough to affect some people adversely. Women with PMS (as well as people with depression, anxiety, insomnia, or any psychological disorder) should avoid caffeine completely.

The combination of caffeine and refined sugar seem to be worse than either substance consumed alone. Several studies have found an association between this combination and depression. In one of the most interesting studies, 21 women and 2 men responded to an advertisement requesting volunteers "who feel depressed and don't know why, often feel tired even though they sleep a lot, are very moody, and generally seem to feel bad most of the time."[20] After baseline psychological testing, the subjects were placed on a caffeine- and sucrose-free diet for one week. Subjects who reported substantial improvement were retested and challenged in a double-blind fash-

Table 7.4   Caffeine Content of Coffee, Tea, and
Selected Soft Drinks

Beverage	Caffeine (mg)
Coffee (7.5 oz cup)	
Drip	115 to 150
Brewed	80 to 135
Instant	65 to 40
Decaffeinated	3 to 4
Tea (5 oz cup)	
1-minute brew	20
3-minute brew	35
Iced (12 oz)	70
Soft drinks	
Jolt	100
Mountain Dew	54
Tab	47
Coca-Cola	45
Diet Coke	45
Dr. Pepper	40
Pepsi Cola	38
Diet Pepsi	36
7 Up	0

ion. The subjects either took a capsule containing caffeine and a Kool-Aid drink sweetened with sugar or they took a capsule containing cellulose and a Kool-Aid drink sweetened with Nutrasweet. Each challenge lasted up to six days. About 50% of the test subjects given caffeine and sucrose became depressed during the test period.

Another study using a similar format found that 7 of 16 depressed patients were found to be depressed with the caffeine and sucrose challenge, but became symptom-free during the caffeine- and sucrose-free diet and cellulose and Nutrasweet test period.[21]

Keeping Your Salt Intake Low

Excessive salt (sodium chloride) consumption, coupled with diminished dietary potassium, greatly stresses the kidney's ability to maintain proper fluid volume. As a result some people are "salt-sensitive" in that high-salt intake causes high blood pressure or, in other cases, water retention. In general, it is a very good idea to avoid salt if you have PMS. If you tend to notice more water retention during the mid-luteal phase, then reducing your salt intake is an absolute must. However, it is simply not a matter of reducing salt intake; you must simultaneously increase your intake of potassium. This is easily done by increasing your intake of high-potassium foods (see Table 7.5) and avoiding high-sodium foods (most processed foods). Read labels carefully and keep your total daily sodium intake below 1,800 mg.

Most Americans have a potassium-to-sodium (K:Na) ratio of less than 1:2. This 1:2 ratio means that most people ingest twice as much sodium as potassium. Yet researchers recommend a dietary potassium-to-sodium ratio of greater than 5:1 to maintain health. This is ten times higher than the average intake. However, even this may not be optimal. A natural diet rich in fruits and vegetables can produce a K:Na ratio greater than 100:1, as most fruits and vegetables have a K:Na ratio of at least 50:1.

If you really must have the taste of salt, try the so-called salt substitutes such as the popular brands NoSalt and Nu-Salt. These products are composed of potassium chloride, which tastes very similar to sodium chloride.

Constructing a Healthful Diet

The American Dietetic Association (ADA) in conjunction with the American Diabetes Association and other groups,

Table 7.5   Potassium/Sodium Content of Selected Foods,
             in Milligrams per Serving

Food	Portion Size	Potassium	Sodium
Fresh Vegetables			
Asparagus	½ cup	165	1
Avocado	½	680	5
Carrot, raw	1	225	38
Corn	½ cup	136	trace
Lima beans, cooked	½ cup	581	1
Potato	1 medium	782	6
Spinach, cooked	½ cup	292	45
Tomato, raw	1 medium	444	5
Fresh Fruits			
Apple	1 medium	182	2
Apricots, dried	¼ cup	318	9
Banana	1 medium	440	1
Cantaloupe	¼ melon	341	17
Orange	1 medium	263	1
Peach	1 medium	308	2
Plums	5	150	1
Strawberries	½ cup	122	trace
Unprocessed Meats			
Chicken, light meat	3 ounces	350	54
Lamb, leg	3 ounces	241	53
Roast beef	3 ounces	224	49
Pork	3 ounces	219	48
Fish			
Cod	3 ounces	345	93
Flounder	3 ounces	498	201
Haddock	3 ounces	297	150
Salmon	3 ounces	378	99
Tuna, drained solids	3 ounces	225	38

has developed the Exchange System, a convenient tool for the rapid estimation of the calorie, protein, fat, and carbohydrate content of a diet. Originally used in designing dietary recommendations for diabetics, the Exchange System is now used in the calculation and design of virtually all therapeutic diets. Unfortunately, the ADA system does not place a strong enough focus on the *quality* of food choices.

The Healthy Exchange System presented here, as well as in *The Healing Power of Foods* (Prima Publishing, 1993), is a superior version because it emphasizes more healthful food choices and focuses on unprocessed, whole foods. The diet is prescribed by allotting the number of exchanges allowed per list for one day. There are seven exchange lists; however, the milk and meat lists should be considered optional:

The Healthy Exchange System

Vegetables

Fruits

Breads, Cereals, and Starchy Vegetables

Legumes

Fats and Oils

Milk

Meats, Fish, Cheese, and Eggs

Because all food portions within each exchange list provide approximately the same calories, proteins, fats, and carbohydrates per serving it is easy to construct a diet consisting of the recommended percentages of:

Carbohydrates:	65% to 75% of total calories
Fats:	15% to 25% of total calories
Protein:	10% to 15% of total calories
Dietary fiber:	at least 50 grams

Of the carbohydrates ingested, 90% should be complex carbohydrates or naturally occurring sugars. Intake of refined carbohydrates and concentrated sugars (including honey, pasteurized fruit juices, dried fruit, sugar, and white flour) should be limited to less than 10% of your total calorie intake.

Constructing a diet that meets these recommendations is simple using the exchange lists. In addition, the recommendations ensure a high intake of vital whole foods, particularly vegetables, rich in nutritional value.

How Many Calories Do You Need?

In determining calorie needs, it is necessary to first determine ideal body weight. The most popular height and weight charts are the tables of "desirable weight" provided by the Metropolitan Life Insurance Company. The most recent edition of these tables, published in 1983, gives weight ranges at one-inch increments of height for three body frame sizes.

Determining Frame Size

To make a simple determination of your frame size: Extend your arm and bend your forearm upward at a 90-degree angle. Keep your fingers straight and turn the inside of your wrist away from your body. Place the thumb and index finger of your other hand on the two prominent bones on either side of your elbow. Measure the space between your fingers with a tape measure. Compare the measurement with the following measurements for medium-framed individuals. A lower reading indicates a small frame; a higher readings indicates a large frame.

Measurements for Medium-Frame Size—Women

Height in 1-inch heels	Elbow breadth
4'10" to 5'3"	2¼ " to 2½"
5'4" to 5'11"	2⅜" to 2⅝"
6'0"	2½" to 2¾"

Table 7.6 1983 Metropolitan Height and Weight Table for Women*

Height	Small Frame	Medium Frame	Large Frame
Women			
4'10"	102–111	109–121	118–131
4'11"	103–113	111–123	120–134
5'0"	104–115	113–126	122–137
5'1"	106–118	115–129	125–140
5'2"	108–121	118–132	128–143
5'3"	111–124	121–135	131–147
5'4"	114–127	124–138	134–151
5'5"	117–130	127–141	137–155
5'6"	120–133	130–144	140–159
5'7"	123–136	133–147	143–163
5'8"	126–139	136–150	146–167
5'9"	129–142	139–153	149–170
5'10"	132–145	142–156	152–173
5'11"	135–148	145–159	155–176
6'0"	138–151	148–162	158–179

*Weights for adults ages 25 to 59 years based on lowest mortality. Weight in pounds according to frame size in indoor clothing (5 pounds for men and 3 pounds for women) wearing shoes with 1-inch heels

After determining your desirable weight in pounds, convert it to kilograms by dividing it by 2.2. Next, take this number and multiply it by the following calories, depending upon activity level:

Little physical activity:	30 calories
Light physical activity:	35 calories
Moderate physical activity:	40 calories
Heavy physical activity:	45 calories

Weight (in Kg) × Activity Level = Approximate Calorie Requirements

_____ × _____ = _____

Examples of Exchange Recommendations

1,500 Calorie Vegan Diet

  Vegetables: 5 servings
  Fruits: 2 servings
  Breads, Cereals, and Starchy Vegetables: 9 servings
  Beans: 2.5 servings
  Fats: 4 servings

The above diet would result in an intake of approximately 1,500 calories per day, of which 67% are derived from complex carbohydrates and naturally occurring sugars, 18% from fat, and 15% from protein. The protein intake is entirely from plant sources, but still provides approximately 55 grams; this number is well above the recommended daily allowance of protein intake for someone requiring 1,500 calories. At least half of the fat servings should be from nuts, seeds, and other whole foods from the fat exchange list. The dietary fiber intake would be approximately 31 to 74.5 grams.

1,500 Calorie Omnivore Diet

  Vegetables: 5 servings
  Fruits: 2.5 servings
  Breads, Cereals, and Starchy Vegetables: 6 servings
  Beans: 1 serving
  Fats: 5 servings
  Milk: 1 serving
  Meats, Fish, Cheese, and Eggs: 2 servings
      Percentage of calories as carbohydrates: 67%
      Percentage of calories as fats: 18%
      Percentage of calories as protein: 15%
      Protein content: 61 g (75% from plant sources)
      Dietary fiber content: 19.5 to 53.5 g

2,000 Calorie Vegan Diet
    Vegetables: 5.5 servings
    Fruits: 2 servings
    Breads, Cereals, and Starchy Vegetables: 11 servings
    Beans: 5 servings
    Fats: 8 servings
        Percentage of calories as carbohydrates: 67%
        Percentage of calories as fats: 18%
        Percentage of calories as protein: 15%
        Protein content: 79 g
        Dietary fiber content: 48.5 to 101.5 g

2,000 Calorie Omnivore Diet
    Vegetables: 5 servings
    Fruits: 2.5 servings
    Breads, Cereals, and Starchy Vegetables: 13 servings
    Beans: 2 servings
    Fats: 7 servings
    Milk: 1 serving
    Meats, Fish, Cheese, and Eggs: 2 servings
        Percentage of calories as carbohydrates: 66%
        Percentage of calories as fats: 19%
        Percentage of calories as protein: 15%
        Protein content: 78 g (72% from plant sources)
        Dietary fiber content: 32.5 to 88.5 g

2,500 Calorie Vegan Diet
    Vegetables: 8 servings
    Fruits: 3 servings
    Breads, Cereals, and Starchy Vegetables: 17 servings
    Beans: 5 servings
    Fats: 8 servings

Percentage of calories as carbohydrates: 69%
Percentage of calories as fats: 15%
Percentage of calories as protein: 16%
Protein content: 101 g
Dietary fiber content: 33 to 121 g

2,500 Calorie Omnivore Diet
Vegetables: 8 servings
Fruits: 3.5 servings
Breads, Cereals, and Starchy Vegetables: 17 servings
Beans: 2 servings
Fats: 8 servings
Milk: 1 serving
Meats, Fish, Cheese, and Eggs: 3 servings
Percentage of calories as carbohydrates: 66%
Percentage of calories as fats: 18%
Percentage of calories as protein: 16%
Protein content: 102 g (80% from plant sources)
Dietary fiber content: 40.5 to 116.5 g

3,000 Calorie Vegan Diet
Vegetables: 10 servings
Fruits: 4 servings
Breads, Cereals, and Starchy Vegetables: 17 servings
Beans: 6 servings
Fats: 10 servings
Percentage of calories as carbohydrates: 70%
Percentage of calories as fats: 16%
Percentage of calories as protein: 14%
Protein content: 116 g
Dietary fiber content: 50 to 84 g

3,000 Calorie Omnivore Diet
  Vegetables: 10 servings
  Fruits: 3 servings
  Breads, Cereals, and Starchy Vegetables: 20 servings
  Beans: 2 servings
  Fats: 10 servings
  Milk: 1 serving
  Meats, Fish, Cheese, and Eggs: 3 servings
      Percentage of calories as carbohydrates: 67%
      Percentage of calories as fats: 18%
      Percentage of calories as protein: 15%
      Protein content: 116 g (81% from plant sources)
      Dietary fiber content: 45 to 133 g

Note: Use these recommendations as the basis for calculating other calorie diets. For example, for a 4,000 calorie diet add the 2,500 to the 1,500. For a 1,000 calorie diet divide the 2,000 calorie diet in half.

The Healthy Exchange Lists

Vegetables

Vegetables provide the broadest range of nutrients of any food class. They are rich sources of vitamins, minerals, carbohydrates, and protein. The little fat they contain is in the form of essential fatty acids. Vegetables provide high quantities of other valuable health-promoting substances, especially fiber and carotenes. In Latin, the word *vegetable* means "to enliven or animate." Vegetables give us life. More and more evidence shows vegetables can prevent as well as treat many diseases.

The best way to consume many vegetables is in their fresh, raw form. In their fresh form, many of the nutrients and health-promoting compounds of vegetables are provided in much higher concentrations. Drinking fresh vegetable juices is a phenomenal way to make sure you are achieving your daily quota of vegetables.

When cooking vegetables it is very important that they not be overcooked. Overcooking will not only result in loss of important nutrients it will also alter the flavor of the vegetable. Light steaming, baking, and quick stir-frying are the best ways to cook vegetables. Do not boil vegetables unless you are making soup, because much of the nutrients will be left in the water. If fresh vegetables are not available, frozen vegetables are preferred over their canned counterparts.

Vegetables are fantastic "diet" foods because they are very high in nutritional value, but low in calories. In the list below you will notice there is also a sublist of "free" vegetables. These vegetables are termed "free foods" and can be eaten in any desired amount because the calories they contain are offset by the number of calories your body burns in the process of digestion. If you are trying to lose weight, these foods are especially valuable as they help to keep you feeling satisfied between meals.

The list below shows the vegetables to use for one vegetable exchange. One cup of cooked vegetables or fresh vegetable juice or 2 cups of raw vegetables equal one exchange. Please notice that starchy vegetables such potatoes and yams are included in the Breads, Cereals, and Starchy Vegetables list below.

Vegetables

    Artichoke (1 medium)

    Asparagus

    Bean sprouts

    Beets

    Broccoli

Brussels sprouts
Carrots
Cauliflower
Eggplant
Greens:
    Beet
    Chard
    Collard
    Dandelion
    Kale
    Mustard
    Spinach
    Turnip
Mushrooms
Okra
Onions
Rhubarb
Rutabaga
Sauerkraut
String beans, green or yellow
Summer squash
Tomatoes, tomato juice, vegetable juice cocktail
Zucchini

Free Vegetables (may be eaten as often as desired, especially in their raw form)
Alfalfa sprouts
Bell peppers
Bok choy
Cabbage

Chicory

Celery

Chinese cabbage

Cucumber

Endive

Escarole

Lettuce

Parsley

Radishes

Spinach

Turnips

Watercress

Fruits

Fruits are a rich source of many beneficial compounds and regular fruit consumption has been shown to offer significant protection against many chronic degenerative diseases including cancer, heart disease, cataracts, and strokes. Fruits make excellent snacks because they contain fructose or fruit sugar, which is absorbed slowly into the bloodstream thereby allowing the body time to utilize it. Fruits are also excellent sources of vitamins and minerals as well as health-promoting fiber compounds. However, fruits are not as nutrient dense as vegetables because they are typically higher in calories. That is why vegetables are favored over fruits in weight-loss plans and overall healthful diets.

If you are a diabetic, be careful to monitor your blood glucose levels after drinking guava, grapefruit, or any other fruit juice because it may necessitate changing the dosage of your medication.

Fruits
Each of the following equals one exchange:

Fresh juice, 1 cup (8 oz)
Pasteurized juice, ⅔ cup
Apple, 1 large
Applesauce (unsweetened), 1 cup
Apricots, fresh, 4 medium
Apricots, dried, 8 halves
Banana, 1 medium
Berries:
    Blackberries, 1 cup
    Blueberries, 1 cup
    Cranberries, 1 cup
    Raspberries, 1 cup
    Strawberries, 1½ cups
Cherries, 20 large
Dates, 4
Figs, fresh, 2
Figs, dried, 2
Grapefruit, 1
Grapes, 20
Mango, 1 small
Melons:
    Cantaloupe, ½ small
    Honeydew, ¼ medium
    Watermelon, 2 cups
Nectarines, 2 small
Orange, 1 large
Papaya, 1½ cups

Peaches, 2 medium

Persimmons, native, 2 medium

Pineapple, 1 cup

Plums, 4 medium

Prunes, 4 medium

Prune juice, ½ cup

Raisins, 4 tbsp

Tangerines, 2 medium

Additional fruit exchanges (no more than one per day):

Honey, 1 tbsp

Jams, jellies, preserves, 1 tbsp

Sugar, 1 tbsp

Breads, Cereals, and Starchy Vegetables

Breads, cereals, and starchy vegetables are classified as complex carbohydrates. Chemically, complex carbohydrates are made up of long chains of simple carbohydrates or sugars, which means that the body has to break down the large sugar chains into simple sugars. Therefore, the sugar from complex carbohydrates enters the bloodstream more slowly than with simple carbohydrates, and blood-sugar levels and appetite are better controlled.

Complex carbohydrates such as breads, cereals, and starchy vegetables are higher in fiber and nutrients and lower in calories than foods high in simple sugars such as cakes and candies. Choose whole grain products (e.g., whole grain breads, whole grain flour products, brown rice, etc.) over their processed counterparts (white bread, white flour products, white rice, etc.). Whole grains provide substantially more nutrients and health-promoting properties. Whole grains are a major source of complex carbohydrates, dietary fiber, minerals, and B vitamins. The protein content and quality of whole grains is greater than that of refined grains. Diets rich in whole grains have been shown to be protective against the development of chronic degenerative diseases, especially cancer, heart disease, diabetes, varicose veins, and diseases of the colon including colon cancer, inflammatory bowel disease, hemorrhoids, and diverticulitis.

Whole grains can be used as breakfast cereals, side dishes, casseroles, or as part of an entree.

Breads, Cereals, and Starchy Vegetables
One of the following equals one exchange:

Breads
Bagel, small, ½
Dinner roll, 1
Dried bread crumbs, 3 tbsp
English muffin, small, ½
Tortilla (6-inch diameter), 1
Whole wheat, rye, or pumpernickel, 1 slice

Cereals
Bran flakes, ½ cup
Cornmeal (dry), 2 tbsp
Cereal (cooked), ½ cup
Flour, 2½ tbsp
Grits (cooked), ½ cup
Pasta (cooked), ½ cup
Puffed cereal (unsweetened), 1 cup
Rice or barley (cooked), ½ cup

Wheat germ, ¼ cup
Other unsweetened cereal, ¾ cup

Crackers
Arrowroot, 3
Graham (2½-inch square), 2
Matzo (4 × 6 inches), ½
Rye wafers (2 × 3½ inches), 3
Saltines, 6

Starchy vegetables
Corn kernels, ⅓ cup
Corn on cob, 1 small
Parsnips, ⅔ cup
Potato, mashed, ½ cup
Potato, baked, 1 small
Squash, winter, ½ cup
Yam or sweet potato, ¼ cup

Prepared foods
Biscuit, 2-inch diameter (omit 1 fat exchange), 1
Corn bread, 2 × 2 × 1 inch (omit 1 fat exchange), 1
French fries, 2 to 3 inches long (omit 1 fat exchange), 8
Muffin, small (omit 1 fat exchange), 1
Potato or corn chips (omit 2 fat exchanges), 15
Pancake, 5 × ½ inch (omit 1 fat exchange), 1
Waffle, 5 × ½ inch (omit 1 fat exchange), 1

Legumes

Legumes (beans) are among the oldest cultivated plants; fossil records demonstrate that even prehistoric people domesticated and cultivated certain legumes for food. Today, legumes are a mainstay in most diets of the world, second only to grains in supplying calories and protein to the world's population. Compared to grains, they supply about the same number of total calories, but they usually provide two to four times as much protein. Legumes are often called the "poor people's meat," however, they might be better known as the "healthy people's meat." Although lacking some key amino acids, when legumes are combined with grains they form what is known as a *complete protein* in that they provide a more complete amino acid profile.

Legumes are fantastic foods, rich in important nutrients and health-promoting compounds. Legumes help improve liver function and lower cholesterol levels and they are extremely effective in improving blood-sugar control.

Legumes and Flatulence   One of the problems with legumes is increased intestinal flatulence (gas) or intestinal discomfort. Most humans pass gas a total of 14 times per day for a total of one pint. About half of the gas is swallowed air and another 40% is carbon dioxide given off by the bacteria in the intestines. The remaining 10% is a mixture of hydrogen, methane, and sulfur compounds as well as byproducts of bacteria. It is this last fraction that is responsible for the offensive odors.

The flatulence-causing compounds in legumes are primarily oligosaccharides, which are composed of three to five sugar molecules linked together in such a way that the body cannot digest or absorb them. Because the body cannot absorb or digest these oligosaccharides, they pass into the intestines where bacteria break them down. Gas is produced by the bacteria as they digest the oligosaccharides. Navy and lima beans are generally the most offensive, while peanuts are the least because of the lower level of these compounds.

The amount of flatulence produced by legumes can be dramatically reduced by properly cooking or sprouting them. A commercial enzyme preparation (Beano) is also available to help reduce flatulence.

Cooking Dried Legumes   Although most legumes can be purchased precooked in cans, cooking your own offers significant economic (buying dried legumes is much cheaper than canned) as well as health benefits (canned legumes can be high in sodium).

Dried legumes are best prepared by first soaking them overnight in four cups of water for every one cup of dried legumes. This is best done in the refrigerator to prevent fermentation. Soaking will usually cut the cooking time dramatically. If soaking overnight is not possible, here is an alternate method:

Place the dried legumes in an appropriate amount of water in a pot (for most legumes this is three cups of water for every one cup of dried legumes). For each cup of dried legumes, add ¼ teaspoon of baking soda, bring to a boil for at least two minutes, and then set aside to soak for at least an hour. The baking soda will soften the legumes and help to break down the troublesome oligo-saccharides. The baking soda will also help reduce the amount of cooking time. After soaking, legumes should be simmered with a minimum of stirring to keep them firm and unbroken. A pressure cooker or Crock-Pot can also be used for convenience.

Sprouting Legumes   Since legumes are actually seeds, they can be sprouted. Sprouting is thought to not only increase the nutritional value for many legumes, it is thought to improve their digestibility as well. Many sprouts, such as alfalfa, mung bean, garbanzo beans, and lentils, are available at grocery stores. Alfalfa sprouts are, by far, the most popular.

Sprouting at home is quite easy for most nuts, seeds, grains, and legumes. All you need is a large glass jar or, better yet, invest in a sprouting jar with different types of lids. After rinsing, place the item to be sprouted in the jar, cover with water for 24 hours. You may need to rinse the item once or twice and re-cover with water. After the initial 24 hours, pour out the water, rinse, and allow the moist sprouts to sit in an area without direct sunlight. Rinse the sprouts twice daily. Once the item has sprouted (usually one to two days) it can be placed in more direct sunlight if desired. Most sprouts will be ready to eat a day or two after they have sprouted.

Legumes
One-half cup of the following cooked or sprouted beans equals one exchange:

   Black-eyed peas

   Garbanzo beans

   Kidney beans

   Lentils

   Lima beans

   Pinto beans

   Soybeans, including tofu (omit 1 fat exchange)

   Split peas

   Other dried beans and peas

Fats and Oils

Saturated fats are known to exert negative effects on glucose control and are linked to both diabetes and hypoglycemia. Saturated fats are typically animal fats and are solid at room temperature. In contrast, vegetable fats are liquid at room temperature and are referred to as unsaturated fats or oils. Our body requires certain oils as essential, specifically, the fatty acids linoleic and linolenic acid. These fatty acids function in our bodies as components of nerve cells, cellular membranes, and hormone-like substances known as prostaglandins. Increased consumption

of essential fatty acids has been shown to lower cholesterol levels and improve many aspects of diabetes.
While essential fatty acids are critical to human health,
too much fat in the diet, especially saturated fat, is linked
to numerous cancers, heart disease, and strokes. It is
strongly recommended by most nutritional experts that
your total fat intake be kept below 30% of the total calories you consume each day. It is also recommended that at
least twice as much unsaturated fats be consumed as saturated fats. This recommendation is easy to follow by
simply reducing the amount of animal products in your
diet, increasing the amount of nuts and seeds consumed,
and using natural polyunsaturated oils.

Most commercially available salad dressings, as well
as those in restaurants, are full of the wrong type of fats
and oils. Salad dressings are the perfect opportunity to use
some of the more polyunsaturated and therapeutic vegetable oils such as flaxseed, safflower, sunflower, and soy.
Flax for Life, by Jade Beutler, is a good source of recipes (to
order, call 1-800-445-3529). I often use:

Basil Dressing

Makes 6 Servings (2 tablespoons per serving)

¼   cup flaxseed oil

3   tablespoons fresh lemon juice

¼   cup water

2   tablespoons minced fresh basil or 1½ teaspoons
dried basil

1   teaspoon finely chopped garlic

Black pepper to taste

Combine all ingredients in a blender or food processor
and mix thoroughly.

Fats and Oils
Each of the following equals one exchange:

Polyunsaturated
Vegetable Oils
    Canola, 1 tsp
    Corn, 1 tsp
    Flaxseed, 1 tsp
    Safflower, 1 tsp
    Soy, 1 tsp
    Sunflower, 1 tsp
Avocado (4-inch diameter), ⅛
Almonds, 10 whole
Pecans, 2 large
Peanuts:
    Spanish, 20 whole
    Virginia, 10 whole
Walnuts, 6 small
Seeds
    Flax, 1 tbsp
    Pumpkin, 1 tbsp
    Sesame, 1 tbsp
    Sunflower, 1 tbsp

Monounsaturated
Olive oil, 1 tsp
Olives, 5 small

Saturated (use sparingly)
Butter, 1 tsp
Bacon, 1 slice

Cream, light or sour, 2 tbsp

Cream, heavy, 1 tbsp

Cream cheese, 1 tbsp

Salad dressings, 2 tsp

Mayonnaise, 1 tsp

Milk

Is milk for "everybody"? Definitely not. Many people are allergic to milk or lack the enzymes necessary to digest milk. The drinking of cow's milk is a relatively new dietary practice for humans. This may be the reason that so many people have difficulty with milk. Women with PMS have been shown to drink more milk than women without PMS. Eliminating milk from the diet altogether has been a popular recommendation by many PMS experts (such as Dr. Guy Abraham).[1] Certainly milk consumption should be limited to no more than one or two servings per day. Choose nonfat products.

Milk and Milk Products
One cup equals one exchange.

Nonfat milk or yogurt

2% milk (omit 1 fat exchange)

Lowfat yogurt (omit 1 fat exchange)

Whole milk (omit 2 fat exchanges)

Whole milk yogurt (omit 2 fat exchanges)

Meats, Fish, Cheese, and Eggs

When choosing from this list, it is important to choose primarily from the lowfat group and remove the skin of poultry. This will keep the amount of saturated fat low. Although many people advocate vegetarianism, the exchange list below provides high concentrations of certain nutrients (such as the full-range of amino acids, vitamin B_{12}, and iron) difficult to get in an entirely vegetarian diet. The most important recommendation may be to use these foods in small amounts as "condiments" in the diet rather than as mainstays. Definitely stay away from cured meats such as bacon, pastrami, and ham because these foods are rich in compounds that can lead to the formation of cancer-causing compounds known as nitrosamines.

Possible exceptions to the recommendation of reducing your intake of animal foods are cold-water fish such as salmon, mackerel, and herring, which provide oils known as omega-3 fatty acids. These beneficial oils have been shown in hundreds of studies to lower cholesterol and triglyceride levels, thereby reducing the risk of heart disease and strokes. The omega-3 fatty acids are not only recommended to treat or prevent high cholesterol levels, but also high blood pressure, other cardiovascular diseases, cancer, auto-immune diseases such as multiple sclerosis and rheumatoid arthritis, allergies and inflammation, eczema, psoriasis, and many other diseases.

Meats, Fish, Cheese, and Eggs
Each of the following equals one exchange:

> *Lowfat (less than 15% fat content)*
> Beef, 1 oz
>> Baby beef, chipped beef, chuck, steak (flank, plate), tenderloin plate ribs, round (bottom, top), all cuts rump, spare ribs, tripe
>
> Cottage cheese, lowfat, ¼ cup
>
> Fish, 1 oz
>
> Lamb, 1 oz
>> Leg, rib, sirloin, loin (roast and chops), shank, shoulder

Poultry (chicken or turkey without skin), 1 oz

Veal, 1 oz

  Leg, loin, rib, shank, shoulder, cutlet

Medium fat (for each omit ½ fat exchange)

Beef, 1 oz

  Ground (15% fat), canned corned beef, rib eye, round (ground commercial)

Cheese, 1 oz

  Mozzarella, ricotta, farmer's, Parmesan

Eggs, 1

Organ meats, 1 oz

Peanut butter, 2 tbsp

Pork, 1 oz

  Loin (all tenderloin), picnic and boiled ham, shoulder, Boston butt, Canadian bacon

High fat (for each exchange omit 1 fat exchange)

Beef, 1 oz

  Brisket, corned beef, ground beef (more than 20% fat), hamburger, roasts (rib), steaks (club and rib)

Cheese, Cheddar, 1 oz

Duck or goose, 1 oz

Lamb breast, 1 oz

Pork, 1 oz

  Spareribs, ground pork, country-style ham, deviled ham

Menu Planning

The Healthy Exchange System was created to ensure that you are consuming a healthful diet that is providing adequate levels of nutrients in their proper ratio. It is important that you have determined your caloric needs and have calculated the number of servings required from each Healthy Exchange List. This will help a great deal when constructing a daily menu.

Breakfast

Breakfast is an absolute must. Healthful breakfast choices include whole grain cereals, muffins, and breads along with fresh whole fruit or fresh fruit juice. Cereals, both hot and cold, and preferably from whole grains, may be the best food choice for breakfast. The complex carbohydrates in grains provide sustained energy. An evaluation of data from the National Health and Nutrition Examination Survey II (a national survey of the nutritional and health practices of Americans) disclosed that serum cholesterol levels are lowest among adults eating whole grain cereal for breakfast.[22] Although those individuals who consumed other breakfast foods had higher blood cholesterol levels, levels were highest among those who typically skipped breakfast.

Lunch

Lunch is a great time to enjoy a healthful bowl of soup, a large salad, and some whole grain bread. Bean soups and other legume dishes are especially good lunch selections for people with diabetes and blood sugar problems, due to their ability to improve blood-sugar regulation. Legumes are filling, yet low in calories.

Dinner

For dinner, the most healthful meals contain a fresh vegetable salad, a cooked vegetable side dish or a bowl of soup, whole grains, and legumes. The whole grains may be provided in bread, pasta, pizza or as a side dish or entree. The legumes can be utilized in soups, salads, and main dishes.

Although a varied diet rich in whole grains, vegetables, and legumes provides optimal levels of protein, some people like to eat meat. The important thing is not to over-consume animal products. Limit your intake to no more than 4 to 6 ounces per day and choose fish, skinless poultry, and lean cuts rather than fat-laden choices.

Final Comments

Many nutrition-oriented physicians believe that food allergies are often responsible for many of the symptoms of PMS. Food allergies refer to an allergic reaction caused by the ingestion of a food. It is estimated by some experts that at least 60% of Americans suffer from negative reactions to food. Food allergies have been shown to be an important cause in a wide range of conditions.

Symptoms and Diseases Commonly Associated with Food Allergy

System	Symptoms and Diseases
Gastrointestinal	Canker sores, celiac disease, chronic diarrhea, stomach ulcer, gas, gastritis, irritable colon, malabsorption, ulcerative colitis
Genitourinary	Bedwetting, chronic bladder infections, kidney disease
Immune	Chronic infections, frequent ear infections

Brain	Anxiety, depression, hyperactivity, inability to concentrate, insomnia, irritability, mental confusion, personality change, seizures
Musculoskeletal	Bursitis, joint pain, low back pain
Respiratory	Asthma, chronic bronchitis, wheezing
Skin	Acne, eczema, hives, itching, skin rash
Miscellaneous	Irregular heart beats, edema, fainting, fatigue, headache, hypoglycemia, itchy nose or throat, migraines, sinusitis

An elimination diet can determine if food allergy is playing a major role in a particular health condition. The standard elimination diet consists of lamb, chicken, rice, banana, apples, and a vegetable from the cabbage family. This diet is also called an *oligoantigenic diet*. After consuming only these foods for a period of at least 10 days, the next step is the reintroduction of foods. A daily record book is necessary so that you can keep a detailed journal of the dates when new foods are introduced and any adverse responses in your body. Every second day a food can be reintroduced to the diet. If the food is one to which an individual is sensitive, the symptoms of the adverse response will reappear (often more strongly than before). The two-day wait before reintroducing the next food allows a period of up to 48 hours where such symptoms will likely be an adverse response to the reintroduced food.

An alternative to the elimination diet is to check for food allergies by blood analysis (the conventional skin scratch test is virtually worthless for food allergies). These tests are convenient, but can range in cost from a modest

$130 to an extravagant $1,200. In my clinical practice, I tend to favor the ELISA tests, which determine both IgE- and IgG-mediated food allergies. Laboratories that I would recommend to perform this analysis are National BioTech Laboratory (1-800-846-6285) and Meridian Valley Clinical Laboratory (1-206-859-8700). These laboratories offer IgE and IgG food allergy panel tests for over 100 different foods, comes with detailed dietary instructions, and are reasonably priced at about $130.

8

Nutritional Supplementation

The key functions of nutrients such as vitamins and minerals revolve around their role as essential components in enzymes and coenzymes in the human body. Enzymes are molecules involved in speeding up chemical reactions necessary for human bodily function. Coenzymes are molecules that help the enzymes in their chemical reactions.

Although all essential nutrients are critical to good health, our discussion in this chapter will focus on the following six key nutrients followed by some practical recommendations:

Vitamin B_6

Magnesium

Calcium

Zinc

Vitamin E

Essential fatty acids

Vitamin B$_6$

The first use of vitamin B$_6$ (pyridoxine) in the management of cyclical conditions in women was in the successful treatment of depression caused by birth control pills in the early 1970s. The results of these studies led researchers to try to determine the effectiveness of vitamin B$_6$ in relieving PMS symptoms. Since 1975 there have been at least a dozen double-blind clinical trials.[1,2] The majority of these studies have demonstrated that vitamin B$_6$ has a positive effect. For example, in one double-blind crossover trial, 84% of the subjects had a lower symptomatology score during the B$_6$ treatment period.[3] Although PMS has multiple causes, B$_6$ supplementation alone appears to benefit most patients.

However, not all double-blind studies of vitamin B$_6$ have been positive.[1,2] The negative results may have been caused by many factors, such as the inability of some women to convert vitamin B$_6$ to its active form due to a deficiency in another nutrient (e.g., vitamin B2 or magnesium), which was not supplemented. Supplementing pyridoxine by itself may not result in adequate clinical results for all women suffering from PMS because some women may have difficulty converting vitamin B$_6$ into its active form, pyridoxal-5-phosphate. To overcome this conversion difficulty, it may be necessary to use a broader-spectrum nutritional supplement or injectable pyridoxal-5-phosphate.

Vitamin B$_6$ Dosage Ranges

For most indications, the therapeutic dosage of vitamin B$_6$ is 50 to 100 mg daily. This dosage level is generally regarded as being safe, even for long-term use. When using dosages greater than 50 mg, it may be important to divide it into 50 mg dosages throughout the day. In a study, a single dosage of 100 mg of pyridoxine did *not* lead to a significant increase in pyridoxal-5-phosphate levels in the blood, indicating that a 50 mg oral dosage of pyridoxine is about all the liver can handle at once.[4]

Safety of Vitamin B*₆*

Vitamin B$_6$ is one of the few water-soluble vitamins that is associated with some toxicity when taken in large or moderate doses for long periods of time. One-time doses greater than 2,000 mg per day can produce symptoms of nerve toxicity (tingling sensations in the feet, loss of muscle coordination, and degeneration of nerve tissue) in some individuals. Chronic intake of doses greater than 500 mg daily can be toxic if taken daily for many months or years.[5] There are also a few rare reports of toxicity occurring at chronic long-term dosages as low as 150 mg a day.[5-7] The supplemental pyridoxine is thought to overwhelm the liver's ability to add a phosphate group to form the active form of vitamin B$_6$ (pyridoxal-5-phosphate). As a result, it is speculated that either pyridoxine is toxic to the nerve cells or it actually acts as an anti-metabolite by binding to pyridoxal-5-phosphate receptors, thereby creating a relative deficiency of vitamin B$_6$. Again, it makes sense to limit dosages to 50 mg at a time. If more than 50 mg a day is desired, then the dosages should be spread out throughout the day.

Vitamin B*₆* and Magnesium Interactions

Vitamin B$_6$ and magnesium interact extensively as they work together in many enzyme systems. One of the ways in which vitamin B$_6$ may improve the symptoms of PMS is by increasing the accumulation of magnesium within the cells of the body.[8] In fact, without vitamin B$_6$, magnesium will not get inside the cell.

Magnesium

Magnesium deficiency is strongly implicated as a causative factor in premenstrual syndrome.[9] Magnesium levels in the red blood cells of PMS patients have been shown to be significantly lower than in normal subjects.[10,11] Because magnesium plays such an integral part in normal cell function, magnesium deficiency may account for the wide-range of symptoms attributed to PMS. Furthermore, magnesium deficiency and PMS share many common features, such as headaches, fatigue, irritability, and poor response to stress, and magnesium supplementation has been shown to be an effective treatment of PMS.[12]

A recent study set out to investigate the association between magnesium and PMS by trying to answer two important questions: (1) Do magnesium measures change as a function of menstrual cycle phase? and (2) Do magnesium measures change across the menstrual cycle differentially in PMS patients and controls? Determinations of plasma, red blood cell (RBC), and mononuclear blood cell (MBC) magnesium were made in 26 women with confirmed PMS and in a control group of 19 women during the follicular, ovulatory, early luteal, and late luteal phases of the menstrual cycle.[13]

The principle findings of the study were as follows: (1) there were no significant differences in plasma magnesium levels in PMS patients compared with controls, nor was there a menstrual cycle effect on plasma magnesium in either group; (2) PMS patients had significantly lower RBC and MBC magnesium concentrations compared to controls; (3) these lower RBC and MBC magnesium concentrations were consistent across the menstrual cycle; and (4) magnesium measures did not correlate with the severity of mood symptoms.

The observation of low RBC magnesium concentrations in PMS patients has now been confirmed by four independent studies. The low MBC magnesium concentrations are also consistent with other studies. As discussed above, the role that magnesium plays in PMS symptomatology is multifactorial due to magnesium's critical roles in cellular metabolism. In general, it is thought that women with PMS have a vulnerability to mood swings during the two weeks before menstruation and that chronic intracellular magnesium depletion serves as a major predisposing factor toward these mood swings.

In addition to emotional instability, magnesium deficiency in PMS is characterized by excessive nervous sensitivity with generalized aches and pains and a lower premenstrual pain threshold. One clinical trial of the effect of magnesium supplementation in PMS showed a reduction of nervousness in 89%, reduction of breast tenderness in 96%, and reduction of weight gain in 95% of the subjects.[10] In another double-blind study, high-dosage magnesium supplementation (360 mg three times daily) was shown to dramatically relieve PMS-related mood changes.[12]

While magnesium has been shown to be effective on its own, even better results may be achieved by combining it with vitamin B_6 and other nutrients. Several studies have shown that when PMS patients are given a multivitamin and mineral supplement containing high doses of magnesium and pyridoxine they experience a tremendous reduction in PMS symptoms.[14,15]

Magnesium Dosage Ranges

Many nutritional experts feel that the ideal intake for magnesium should be based on body weight (6 mg per 2.2 pounds body weight). Thus, for a 110-pound person the recommendation would be 300 mg daily, for a 154-pound person 420 mg, and for a 200-pound person 540 mg. For most people I recommend supplementing their diet with additional magnesium in this manner, however, in the treatment of magnesium deficiency or PMS, I will usually recommend twice this amount—12 mg per 2.2 pounds body weight.

Available Forms of Magnesium

Magnesium is available in several different forms. In general, all forms are equally absorbed. However, I prefer magnesium bound to aspartate or the Krebs cycle intermediates (malate, succinate, fumarate, and citrate) over magnesium oxide, gluconate, sulfate, and chloride. Absorption studies indicate that magnesium is easily absorbed orally, especially when it is bound to citrate (and presumably aspartate and other members of the Krebs cycle).[16,17] In addition, magnesium bound to aspartate or Krebs cycle intermediates may also help fight off fatigue (discussed below). Aspartate feeds into the Krebs cycle, the final common pathway for the conversion of glucose, fatty acids, and amino acids to chemical energy (ATP), while citrate, fumarate, malate, and succinate are actual components of Krebs cycle. Evidence suggests that minerals chelated (bound) to the Krebs cycle intermediates are better absorbed, utilized, and tolerated compared to inorganic or relatively insoluble mineral salts including magnesium chloride, oxide, or carbonate. In addition, while inorganic magnesium salts often cause diarrhea at higher dosages, organic forms of magnesium generally do not.

In most cases, I prefer using a balanced mineral formula rather than isolated mineral chelates. When any single mineral is taken at high doses it can impair the absorption of other important minerals. To achieve the recommended level of magnesium for example, I will first check the value in the patient's multiple vitamin and mineral formula. If the level of magnesium is below their needs, I will usually prescribe a multiple mineral formula to achieve the proper levels of magnesium rather than simply prescribing additional magnesium. However, there are some cases where I will use additional magnesium or products containing primarily magnesium. Examples of these cases include angina, congestive heart failure, migraine headaches, and recurrent kidney stones. Again, in all of these conditions I prefer using magnesium bound to Krebs cycle intermediates.

Calcium

Calcium is a bit of a double-edged sword in PMS. High calcium intake due to high milk consumption is linked as a possible causative factor of PMS, perhaps by the combination of calcium, vitamin D, and phosphorus in milk reducing the absorption of magnesium.[10] At the same time, there are studies showing positive improvements in PMS symptomatology with calcium supplementation (1,000 mg to 1,336 mg).[18,19] In one of the more recent studies, calcium and manganese supplementation (1,336 mg and 5.6 mg, respectively) improved mood, concentration, and behavior. In another study, 1,000 mg of calcium per day improved mood and water retention.[18] It is theorized, based primarily on animal research, that calcium improves the altered hormonal patterns, neurotransmitter levels, and smooth muscle responsiveness noted in PMS.

Further support for the importance of calcium supplementation in PMS was the finding that women with PMS have reduced bone mineral density, which increases their risk of osteoporosis[20] Given the importance of calcium (as well as magnesium) to healthy bones, I recommend supplementation of at least 600 mg calcium and 300 mg magnesium regardless of whether or not a woman is experiencing PMS.

Zinc

Zinc levels have been shown to be lower in women with PMS than in those without.[21] Zinc is required for the proper action of many hormones, including sex hormones, as well as in the control of the secretion of hormones. In particular, zinc serves as one of the control factors for prolactin secretion.[22] When zinc levels are low, prolactin release is promoted; when zinc levels are high, prolactin release is inhibited. Hence, when prolactin levels are elevated, as is common in cases of PMS, zinc supplementation is an absolute must.

The dosage range for zinc supplementation for general health support is 15 to 20 mg per day. Since the average American consumes about 10 mg of zinc per day, supplementing an additional 15 to 20 mg results in a daily intake of 25 to 30 mg for most people. When zinc supplementation is being used to address specific needs such as elevated prolactin levels in women, the dosage range is 30 to 45 mg. The better forms of zinc are zinc bound to picolinate, citrate, or monomethionine.

Vitamin E

Although research concerning vitamin E and PMS has focused primarily on its effect on reducing breast tenderness, significant reduction of other PMS symptomatology has also been demonstrated in double-blind studies.[10,23] Nervous tension, headache, fatigue, depression, and insomnia were all significantly reduced with vitamin E supplementation. In one double-blind study, patients receiving vitamin E (400 IU daily) demonstrated a 33% reduction in physical symptoms (such as weight gain and breast tenderness), a 38% reduction in anxiety, and a 27% reduction in depression after three months of use. In contrast, the placebo group only reported a 14% reduction in physical symptoms. The group taking vitamin E also noted higher energy levels, fewer headaches, and less cravings for sweets.[23]

A good dosage for vitamin E is 400 IU per day. Make sure that the vitamin E is a natural form. Natural forms of vitamin E are designated *d-,* as in d-alpha-tocopherol, while synthetic forms are *dl-,* as in dl-alpha-tocopherol. Although the l form has antioxidant activity, it may actually inhibit the d-form from entering cell membranes. Therefore, natural vitamin E (the d form) has greater benefit than the synthetic (dl). My recommendation is to avoid synthetic vitamin E.

Natural Forms	*Synthetic Forms*
d-alpha-tocopherol	dl-alpha-tocopherol
d-alpha-tocopheryl acetate	dl-alpha-tocopheryl acetate
d-alpha-tocopheryl succinate	dl-alpha-tocopheryl succinate

Essential Fatty Acids

The human body cannot function properly without two essential polyunsaturated fats—linoleic and alpha-linolenic acid. Linoleic acid is designated an omega-6 fatty acid because the first unsaturated bond appears at the 6th carbon while alpha-linolenic acid is an omega-3 fatty acid because its first unsaturated bond occurs at the 3rd carbon.

It is estimated by many experts that approximately 80% of our population consumes an insufficient quantity of essential fatty acids. This dietary insufficiency presents a serious health threat to Americans. In addition to providing the body with energy, the essential fatty acids function in our bodies as components of nerve cells, cellular membranes, and hormonelike substances known as *prostaglandins.* Prostaglandins and the essential fatty acids are important in a variety of bodily functions including:

• Steroid production and hormone synthesis
• Regulating pressure in the eyes, joints, and blood vessels
• Regulating response to pain, inflammation, and swelling
• Mediating immune response
• Regulating bodily secretions and their viscosity
• Dilating or constricting blood vessels
• Regulating collateral circulation
• Directing endocrine hormones to their target cells
• Regulating smooth muscle and autonomic reflexes
• Regulating the rate at which cells divide (mitosis)
• Maintaining the fluidity and rigidity of cellular membranes (of which they are primary constituents)
• Regulating the in-flow and out-flux of substances into and out of cells
• Transporting oxygen from red blood cells to body tissues
• Regulating kidney function and fluid balance
• Keeping saturated fats mobile in the bloodstream
• Preventing blood cells from clumping together (conglomeration—the cause of atherosclerotic plaque and blood clots, a cause of stroke)

- Mediating the release of pro-inflammatory substances from cells that may trigger allergic conditions
- Regulating nerve transmission
- Stimulating steroid production
- Providing the primary energy source for the heart muscle

In addition to their critical role in normal physiology, essential fatty acids have been shown to be protective and therapeutic against heart disease, cancer, auto-immune diseases such as multiple sclerosis and rheumatoid arthritis, skin diseases, and many others. These links are well-established in the medical literature, but relatively unknown by the conventional medical community. Over 60 health conditions have now been shown to benefit from essential fatty acid supplementation.[24]

Recognizing Essential Fatty Acid Deficiency

The signs and symptoms of essential fatty acid deficiency may range from mild fatigue to fatal heart attack. Most orthodox health care practitioners may never make the association between a health symptom and essential fatty acid deficiency, therefore the underlying cause of illness will ultimately continue to manifest. Most physicians are not trained in nutrition to begin with and the laboratory analysis to measure essential fatty acid deficiency is not widely available or appreciated. In addition, the symptoms of essential fatty acid deficiency are not as obvious as many other nutrient deficiencies, although the consequences can be deadly. And even if an essential fatty acid deficiency is recognized, few traditional medical doctors know how to treat it.

In general, the symptoms of a deficiency of essential fatty acids can be so vague and broad that they are typically

Table 8.1 Signs and Symptoms Typical of
Essential Fatty Acid Deficiency

Fatigue, malaise, lacking energy	Frequent colds and sickness
Lack of endurance	Aching sore joints
Dry skin	Angina, chest pain
Cracked nails	Depression
Dry lifeless hair	Lack of motivation
Dry mucous membranes, tear ducts, mouth, vagina	Forgetfulness
	High blood pressure
Maldigestion, gas, bloating	History of cardiovascular
Constipation	disease
Immune weakness	Arthritis

written off as one of a myriad of other causes. Suffice it to say, surveys suggest that Americans are up to 90% deficient in the essential fatty acids.[24] In other words, we are only obtaining about 10% of what we need for optimal health. For this reason, I strongly recommend flaxseed oil to all of my patients, regardless of their condition.

Essential Fatty Acids and Prostaglandin Levels in PMS

Women with PMS exhibit essential fatty acid and prostaglandin abnormalities, with a decrease in gamma-linolenic acid (GLA) as the abnormality most often being reported.[25] Gamma-linolenic acid is derived from linolenic acid. This conversion also requires adequate vitamin B_6, magnesium, and zinc levels because these nutrients function in the key enzyme responsible for this conversion—delta-6-desaturase. Given the fact that deficiency of one or more of these nutrients is common in PMS, decreased GLA levels could almost be expected.

GLA Supplements

Evening primrose, black currant, and borage oils contain GLA, with typical levels being 9%, 12%, and 22%, respectively. Although these essential fatty acid sources are quite popular, the research on GLA supplements is controversial and not as convincing as the research on omega-3 oils for most health conditions. In general, given all the benefits of omega-3 fatty acids, I recommend flaxseed oil over GLA supplements, although the formula that I use in my practice (Doctor's Choice Flax Oil Plus) does provide 325 mg of GLA per tablespoon (equal to about six 500 mg capsules of evening primrose oil; the ratio of omega-3 fatty acids to omega-6 fatty acids in the product is 2:1 in favor of the omega-3 oil).

The double-blind studies of the effects of GLA supplements (such as evening primrose oil) in treating PMS are largely negative in that the supplements showed no greater benefit than a placebo. A meta-analysis of the clinical trials of evening primrose oil concluded that it is of little value in the management of PMS. The three most well-controlled studies failed to show any beneficial effects for evening primrose oil.[26-29]

A better approach to correcting the essential fatty acid and prostaglandin abnormalities of PMS is to provide the necessary nutrients required for proper essential fatty acid *metabolism* along with adequate levels of the essential fatty acids and GLA. In other words, it may be more appropriate to provide a broader range of support than simply trying to increase GLA levels.

Anticancer Benefits of Flaxseed Oil

Breast cancer is a major concern for American women as current estimates are that one out of every eight women

Figure 8.1   Prostaglandin metabolism.

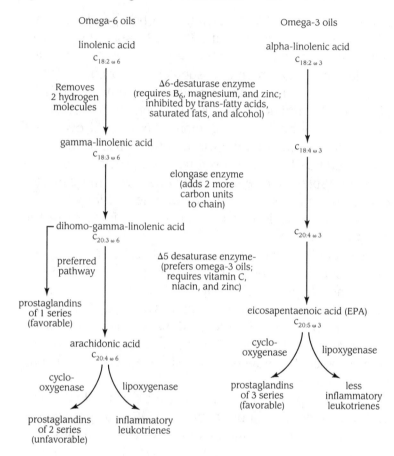

will develop breast cancer in their lifetime. As a result there is increased research on what dietary factors can significantly reduce the risk. In 1990 the National Cancer Institute (NCI) launched a five-year, $20-million program to learn more about biologically active plant chemicals (phytochemicals) in certain foods that may help to prevent cancer. Flaxseed was the first of six foods to be studied. Preliminary results indicated that flaxseed oil can exert powerful anticancer properties, especially against breast cancer. Unfortunately, despite the promise of incredible preliminary results, the NCI project was canceled before it could be completed. Nonetheless, a substantial body of evidence indicates that flaxseed oil exerts significant anticancer properties.

In addition to their high level of alpha-linolenic acid, flaxseeds are the most abundant source of lignans. Lignans are special compounds that are demonstrating some impressive health benefits including positive effects in relieving menopausal hot flashes, as well as anticancer, antibacterial, antifungal, and antiviral activity.

Perhaps the most significant of these actions are the anticancer effects. Population studies, as well as experimental studies in humans and animals, have demonstrated that lignans exert significant anticancer effects.[30–32]

In the animal experiments, tremendous anticancer effects were noted when the animals were fed flaxseeds and flaxseed oil. Positive effects have been shown not only against mammary cancer, but also in colon cancer and general tumor models. Typically, the animals receiving flaxseed oil or flaxseeds demonstrate significant reduction (e.g., greater than 50% reduction) in tumor numbers and size after one to two months.[30–32]

Plant lignans are changed by the gut flora into *enterolactone* and *enterodiol*, two compounds that are believed to be protective against cancer, particularly breast cancer.[33] Like soy phytoestrogens, lignans are capable of binding to estrogen receptors and interfering with the cancer-promoting effects of estrogen on breast tissue. In addition, lignans increase the production of a special sex-hormone binding compound. This compound, known as sex-hormone binding globulin, regulates estrogen levels by escorting excess estrogen from the body via eliminative pathways.

Lignans are thought to be one of the protective factors against breast cancer in vegetarian women.[34] Typically, women who excrete higher amounts of lignans in their urine (a sign of increased consumption) have much lower rates for breast cancer. High-lignan flaxseed oil may be the best choice for women going through menopause or those at risk for breast cancer. It is currently estimated that as many as one in seven American women will develop breast cancer in their lifetime.

Alpha-Linolenic Acid and Breast Cancer

In addition to lignans, a high-lignan flaxseed oil also provides alpha-linolenic acid. Like lignans, alpha-linolenic acid has demonstrated significant anticancer properties, especially against breast cancer. A prospective study in 121 women with initially localized breast cancer examined the association between the levels of various fatty acids in the fatty tissue of the breast and how much the cancer had spread (metastasized).[35] Breast tissue analyzed at the time of surgery indicated that a low level of alpha-linolenic acid was associated with the spread of the cancer into the lymph nodes of the armpit (axillary area) as well as tumor invasiveness.

After 31 months of follow-up after the initial surgery, 21 patients developed metastases of their cancer into other body tissues. Low levels of alpha-linolenic acid were the first determinant of metastases in these patients. In other words, when all factors were considered, low levels of alpha-linolenic acid were found to be the most significant contributor to the spread of cancer. Since the main cause of death in breast cancer patients is the development of cancer in other tissues, this finding is of extreme importance.[36]

The results from this study suggest that supplementing the diet with flaxseed oil (approximately 58% alpha-linolenic acid) may help to prevent breast cancer, tumor invasiveness, and metastasis.

Some Practical Recommendations

I have three primary recommendations for nutritional supplementation in the treatment of PMS:

1. Take a high-quality multiple vitamin and mineral supplement.
2. Take additional antioxidants.
3. Take one tablespoon of flaxseed oil daily.

Multiple Vitamin and Mineral Supplements

Taking a high-quality multiple vitamin and mineral supplement that provides all of the known vitamins and minerals serves a foundation upon which to build. For women with PMS there are two very sound reasons for taking a high-potency multiple supplement:

1. Nutritional deficiency is relatively common among women with PMS.
2. High-potency multiple vitamin and mineral formulations have been shown to produce significant benefits in the treatment of PMS.

The frequency of nutritional supplementation and the intake of selected nutrients by PMS patients has been shown to be much lower than that of women without PMS. Although women with PMS have been shown to consume vitamins in their food at levels that are close to the Recommended Daily Allowance, compared to women who did not have PMS their intake levels were only 2.2% as much for thiamin, 2.2% for riboflavin, 16.7% for niacin, 8.7% for pantothenic acid, and 2.7% for pyridoxine.[10]

Several double-blind studies have shown when PMS patients are given a multiple vitamin and mineral supplement

Table 8.2   Recommended Ranges for Supplemental Vitamins
and Minerals

Vitamins	Range for Adults
Vitamin A (retinol)	2,500 IU
Note: Women of child-bearing age should not take more than 2,500 IU of retinol daily due to the possible risk of birth defects if becoming pregnant is a possibility.	
Vitamin A (from beta-carotene)	5,000–25,000 IU
Vitamin D	100–400 IU
Vitamin E (d-alpha tocopherol)	400–800 IU
Note: It may be more cost-effective to take vitamin E separately.	
Vitamin K (phytonadione)	60–300 mcg
Vitamin C (ascorbic acid)	500–1,500 mg
Note: It may be easier to take vitamin C separately.	
Vitamin B1 (thiamin)	10–100 mg
Vitamin B2 (riboflavin)	10–50 mg
Niacin	10–100 mg
Niacinamide	10–30 mg
Vitamin B$_6$ (pyridoxine)	25–150 mg
Biotin	100–300 mcg
Pantothenic acid	25–100 mg
Folic acid	400 mcg
Vitamin B$_{12}$	400 mcg
Choline	10–100 mg
Inositol	10–100 mg

containing high doses of magnesium and pyridoxine, they experience reductions in (typically at least a 70% reduction) both pre- and post-menstrual symptoms.[14,15]

Table 8.2 lists the daily dosage range recommendations for supplemental vitamins and minerals.

Additional Antioxidants

The two primary antioxidants in the human body are vitamin C and vitamin E. Vitamin C is an *aqueous-phase* anti-

Table 8.2 Recommended Ranges for Supplemental Vitamins and Minerals *(continued)*

Minerals	Range for Adults
Boron	1–6 mg
Calcium	250–1,250 mg

Note: Taking a separate calcium supplement may be necessary when trying to achieve higher dosage levels in women at risk for or suffering from osteoporosis.

Chromium	200–400 mcg

For diabetes and weight loss, dosages of 600 mcg can be used.

Copper	1–2 mg
Iodine	50–150 mcg
Iron	15–30 mg
Magnesium	250–500 mg
Manganese	10–15 mg
Molybdenum	10–25 mcg
Potassium	200–500 mg
Selenium	100–200 mcg
Silica	1–25 mg
Vanadium	50–100 mcg
Zinc	15–45 mg

oxidant, which means that it is found in body compartments composed of water. In contrast, vitamin E is a *lipid-phase* antioxidant because it is found in fat-soluble body compartments, such as cell membranes and fatty molecules. If you are taking a high-potency multiple vitamin and mineral formula, many of the supportive antioxidant nutrients such as selenium, zinc, and beta-carotene are provided for. Therefore, your primary concern in supplementing for additional antioxidants may be simply to ensure that your body obtains beneficial levels of vitamin C and vitamin E. Here are my daily supplementation guidelines for these key nutritional antioxidants for supporting general health. Be sure to recognize how much your multiple vitamin and mineral formula is providing.

Vitamin E (d-alpha tocopherol)   400 to 800 IU

Vitamin C (ascorbic acid) 500 to 1,500 mg

Flaxseed Oil Daily

Organic, unrefined flaxseed oil is considered by many to be the answer to restoring the body's proper level of essential fatty acids. Flaxseed oil is unique because it contains both alpha-linolenic (an omega-3 fatty acid) and linoleic acid (an omega-6 fatty acid) in appreciable amounts. For PMS, I prefer to use a product such as Doctor's Choice Flax Oil Plus, which provides a 2:1 ratio of omega-3 to omega-6, is fortified with lignans, and contains borage oil to provide 325 mg of GLA per tablespoon.

Final Comments

The human body has remarkable homeostatic control mechanisms. *Homeostasis* refers to the body's attempt to maintain a properly balanced internal environment. Homeostatic control mechanisms function in many ways similar to a thermostat in a home. Let's say that your home thermostat is set for a range of 70 to 74 degrees Fahrenheit. When the temperature gets below 70 degrees, the heat kicks on to raise the temperature to the proper range. If the temperature gets above 74 degrees, the air conditioner kicks in. The human body controls its internal environment as well and proper nutrition is absolutely essential in this process. In fact, one of the most beneficial aspects of proper nutritional supplementation is that it helps the body's attempt to maintain homeostasis. In the treatment of PMS, it is important to supplement with a high-quality multiple vitamin and mineral supplement, additional antioxidants, and flaxseed oil daily in order to avoid the nutritional deficiencies that can exacerbate PMS.

Herbal Support for PMS

Although a wide variety of herbs have been used in folk medicine for the many disorders of menstruation and many have been evaluated for their *phytoestrogen* effects, few have been specifically evaluated for their efficacy in relieving premenstrual symptoms. The herbs that are most likely to be useful are probably those which exhibit a tonic effect on the female glandular system. This tonic effect is thought to be a result of phytoestrogens or other compounds in the plants that help to improve the hormonal balance of the female system as well as improving blood flow to the female organs.

Remember, as discussed earlier in this book, phytoestrogens are capable of exerting estrogenic effects, although their activity compared to estrogen is only 2% as strong at the very most. However, because of this low activity, phytoestrogens have a balancing action on estrogen. If estrogen levels are low, since phytoestrogens have some estrogenic activity, they will cause an increase in estrogen effect. If estrogen levels are high, since phytoestrogens bind to estrogen-receptor binding sites, thereby competing with estrogen, there will be a decrease in estrogen effects.

Because of the balancing action of phytoestrogens on estrogen effects, it is common to find the same plant recommended for conditions of estrogen excess (such as PMS) as for conditions of estrogen deficiency (such as menopause and menstrual abnormalities). Many of these herbs have been termed *uterine tonics* because they work to nourish and tone the female glandular and organ system rather than exert a druglike effect.

The four most useful herbs in the treatment of PMS (as well as menopause) are angelica or dong quai (*Angelica sinensis*), licorice root (*Glycyrrhiza glabra*), black cohosh (*Cimicifuga racemosa*), and chaste berry (*Vitex agnuscastus*). These herbs have been used historically to alleviate a variety of female complaints, including hot flashes.

Angelica or Dong Quai

In Asia, angelica's reputation is perhaps second only to ginseng. Predominantly regarded as a "female" remedy, angelica has been used in the treatment of menopausal symptoms (especially hot flashes), as well as in such conditions as dysmenorrhea (painful menstruation), amenorrhea (absence of menstruation), metrorrhagia (abnormal menstruation), and to assure a healthy pregnancy and easy delivery.

Angelica has demonstrated good uterine tonic activity, causing an initial increase in uterine contraction followed by relaxation.[1] Administration of angelica to mice resulted in an increase of uterine weight and increase of glucose utilization by the liver and uterus, effects which reflect phytoestrogenic activities.[2] Angelica is particularly helpful if in addition to PMS a woman experiences painful menstruation.

When using angelica to treat PMS, I generally recommend that it be taken beginning 14 days after the first day of menstruation and continued until the next menstruation. However, if the patient typically experiences dysmenorrhea, I recommend that angelica be continued until menstruation has stopped. Dosage to be taken three times per day:

> Powdered root or as tea, 1 to 2 g
>
> Tincture (1:5), 4 ml (1 tsp)
>
> Fluid extract, 1 ml (¼ tsp)

Licorice Root

The medicinal use of licorice in both Western and Eastern cultures dates back several thousand years. In addition to being used for a variety of female disorders, it was used to alleviate respiratory tract infections and asthma. Its other traditional uses include treating peptic ulcers, malaria, abdominal pain, insomnia, and infections. Many of these uses have been substantiated by modern research.

Licorice is particularly useful in treating PMS because it lowers estrogen levels while raising progesterone levels.[3,4] Licorice raises progesterone levels by inhibiting the enzyme responsible for breaking it down. Licorice may also be useful in reducing water retention.

Remember, aldosterone is the hormone responsible for reducing sodium excretion and, as a result, high levels lead to water retention (edema). Licorice works to block the effects of aldosterone much in the way it impacts estrogen.[5,6] Its chief component, glycyrrhetinic acid, binds to aldosterone receptors but its activity is only about one-quarter as strong as the body's own aldosterone. This lower level of activity means that in cases of high aldosterone levels (such as occurs often in PMS), licorice may reduce the aldosterone effect by competing with aldosterone for binding sites. However, if aldosterone levels are normal, the chronic ingestion of licorice in large doses may cause symptoms of aldosterone excess, namely high blood pressure due to sodium and water retention. It may be possible to prevent the side effects of glycyrrhizin by following a high-potassium, low-sodium diet. Although no formal trial has been performed, patients who normally consume high-potassium foods and restrict their sodium intake, even those with high blood pressure and angina, have been reported to be free from the aldosterone-like side effects of glycyrrhizin.[7] Licorice should probably not be used in patients with a history of hypertension, renal failure, or current use of digitalis preparations.

To treat PMS, I would recommend starting licorice 14 days after the first day of the menstrual cycle and continuing till the next menstruation. Here are dosage recommendations for the various forms of licorice to be taken three times per day:

Powdered root or as tea, 1 to 2 g

Fluid extract (1:1), 4 ml (1 tsp)

Solid (dry powdered) extract (4:1), 250 to 500 mg

Black Cohosh

Black cohosh was widely used by the American Indians and later by American colonists for the relief of menstrual cramps and menopause. Recent scientific investigation on Remifemin (a special extract of black cohosh standardized to contain 1 mg of triterpenes calculated as 27-deoxyacteine per tablet, which has been used in Germany for over 40 years) has shown that it is a safe and effective natural alternative to hormone replacement therapy in the treatment of menopause and may offer some benefits in the treatment of PMS as well.

In the treatment of menopause, several double-blind studies have shown Remifemin to actually produce better results compared to estrogens in several of the studies, especially for hot flashes, atrophic vaginitis, and depression.[8-11] In one double-blind study of 80 menopausal women, Remifemin produced better results than conjugated estrogens (like Premarin) or placebo in all menopausal symptoms, especially hot flashes and atrophic vaginitis.[11] The number of hot flashes experienced each day dropped from an average of 5 to less than 1 in the Remifemin group after 12 weeks. In comparison, the estrogen group only dropped from 5 to 3.5. Even more impressive was the effect of Remifemin on the vaginal lining. While conjugated estrogens as well as the placebo produced little effect, a dramatic increase in the number of superficial cells was noted in the Remifemin group.

In short, while there is significant risk with hormone replacement therapy, Remifemin has been shown to produce symptomatic relief comparable to or better than that of hormone replacement therapy without the risk of serious side effects.

Remifemin has also been reported to be of benefit in the treatment of PMS. In one study of 135 women, Remifemin was judged to have reduced feelings of depression, anxiety, tension, and mood swings.[12]

The usual dosage for menopause is two tablets twice daily (4 mg of 27-deoxyacteine daily); for PMS the dosage is one tablet once or twice daily providing a daily dosage of two to four mg of 27-deoxyacteine.

Chaste Berry

The chaste tree (*Vitex agnus-castus*) is native to the Mediterranean and its berries have long been used to treat female complaints. As its name signifies, chaste berries were used in suppressing the libido.

While Remifemin is the most popular herbal approach to treating menopausal symptoms in Germany, chaste berry extract is probably the most popular herbal approach in the treatment of PMS. In two surveys of gynecological practices in Germany, physicians graded chaste berry extract as good or very good in the treatment of PMS. More than 1,500 women participated in the studies.[13,14] One-third of the women experienced complete resolution of their symptoms after an average treatment length of 166 days, while another 57% reported significant improvement (that is, 90% of the women reported improvement or resolution).

Chaste berry extract appears to be particularly useful in treating cases of corpus luteum insufficiency (see page 5) or prolactin excess.[15] Its beneficial effects on PMS and these other conditions appear to be related to altering the gonadotropin-releasing hormone (GnRH) and follicle-stimulating hormone-releasing hormone (FSH-RH). In other words, it appears that chaste berry extract has profound effects on the hypothalamus and pituitary function. As a result it is able to normalize the secretion of other hormones, such as reducing the secretion of prolactin, and thus reduces the estrogen to progesterone ratio.

Chaste berry extract may be useful in treating certain cases of amenorrhea (absence of menstruation) due to prolactin excess—one of the most frequent causes of amenorrhea. Don't expect immediate results, it takes about three months for chaste berry extract to lower prolactin levels.[15]

The usual dosage of chaste berry extract (often standardized to contain 0.5% agnuside) in tablet or capsule form is 175 to 225 mg daily. If using the liquid extract, the typical dosage is 2 ml daily.

Final Comments

While the above-mentioned herbs are effective individually (especially when being used for well-defined indications, e.g., chaste berry in prolactin excess, licorice in aldosterone excess, angelica when dysmenorrhea is a factor, and black cohosh for menopause), many herbal practitioners often combine them in the belief that greater benefit will be produced. Most major suppliers of herbal products feature formulas containing combinations of these herbs. If using "combination" therapy, I encourage you to use well-respected brands and follow the dosage instructions on the label.

10

Other Female Conditions Associated with PMS

FIBROCYSTIC BREAST DISEASE,
UTERINE FIBROIDS, ENDOMETRIOSIS,
AND CHRONIC CANDIDIASIS

This chapter will provide concise information on four female conditions often associated with PMS—fibrocystic breast disease, uterine fibroids, endometriosis, and chronic candidiasis.

Fibrocystic Breast Disease

Fibrocystic breast disease (FBD), also known as cystic mastitis, is a benign cystic swelling of the breasts. It can be mildly uncomfortable to severely painful, is typically cyclic, and usually precedes a woman's menses. It is the most frequent disease of the breast.

FBD is very common, affecting 20% to 40% of pre-menopausal women. It is usually a component of PMS and is considered a risk factor for breast cancer. It is not, however, as significant a factor as the classic breast-cancer risk factors, i.e., family history, early menarche, and late or no first pregnancy.

Causes of Fibrocystic Breast Disease

Like PMS, the development of FBD is apparently due to an increased estrogen to progesterone ratio. During each menstrual cycle, there is a recurring hormonal stimulation of the breast. As the hormone levels fall, after a few days the breasts normally return to their pre-stimulation size and function. In many women these changes are so slight that clinical signs or symptoms do not appear. In others, however, significant inflammatory processes occur.

The cells of a fibrocystic breast are characterized by overgrowth and enlargement, increased secretory activity, dilation of the milk ducts, and scarring. These effects may be due to increased levels of the hormone prolactin as a result of increased estrogen levels.[1,2]

Treating Fibrocystic Breast Disease

The treatment of FBD is virtually identical to the treatment of PMS. In particular it is especially important to:

Eliminate caffeine and other methylxanthines

Follow the dietary recommendations in Chapter 7

Follow the guidelines for nutritional supplementation in Chapter 8

Rule out low thyroid function

Consider chaste berry extract for herbal support

Caffeine Intake   Strong evidence supports an association between consumption of methylxanthines (caffeine, theophylline, and theobromine) as found in coffee, tea, cola, chocolate, and caffeinated medications (e.g., Excedrin) and FBD.[3-6] Caffeine, theophylline, and theobromine are known to stimulate overproduction of cellular products, such as fibrous tissue and cyst fluid.[4-6] Caffeine has also been implicated in breast cancer.[7]

In one study of FBD, limiting methylxanthines in the diet resulted in improvement in 97.5% of the 45 women who completely abstained and in 75% of the 28 who limited their consumption of coffee, tea, cola, chocolate, and caffeinated medications. Those who continued with little change in their methylxanthine consumption showed little improvement.[4] According to this study, women may have varying thresholds of response to methylxanthines.

Hypothyroidism and Iodine   Hypothyroidism and iodine deficiency are associated with a higher incidence of breast cancer. There is evidence of an association between low thyroid function and FBD as well. Thyroid hormone replacement therapy in hypothyroid, and some normal thyroid, women with FBD may result in improvement. Research has shown that thyroid supplementation decreases breast pain, serum prolactin levels, and breast nodules in patients with supposedly normal thyroids.[8] These results suggest that unrecognized hypothyroidism and/or iodine deficiency may be a causative factor in FBD.

Experimental iodine deficiency in rats results in mammary changes similar on the cellular level to human FBD. It is theorized that an absence of iodine renders the breast tissue more sensitive to estrogen stimulation. This hypersensitivity can produce excess secretions over the limit of absorption, thus distending the breast ducts to produce small cysts and later fibrosis (hardening of the tissue due to the deposition of fibrin similar to the formation of scar tissue). This indicates that iodine may be very important in the treatment and prevention of FBD.

The term *iodine* is commonly used to describe any iodine compound. Technically speaking, only the elemental form of iodine should be referred to as iodine. Iodine complexed to sodium or potassium (the most common supplement form of iodine), is more accurately referred to as an *iodide*. The body appears to handle iodide and iodine differently. Iodides exert a stronger effect on thyroid function. In contrast, elemental iodine appears to be primarily involved in functions outside the thyroid such as the modulation of estrogen action on breast tissue. The reason for this difference is that, unlike thyroid tissue, breast tissue lacks the enzymes which oxidize iodide to iodine. Thus, breast tissue requires elemental forms of iodine. Organic sources of iodine (kelp, iodine caseinate, etc.) are preferred.

Human studies also indicate that elemental iodine is more effective than iodides in the treatment of FBD. Since 1975 three clinical trials have been performed on women with FBD.[9] Results from these studies indicate that while treatment with iodides was effective in about 70% of subjects, it also was associated with a high rate of side effects (e.g., altered thyroid function in 4%, iodism [a condition of iodine excess characterized by extreme weakness, acne-like skin lesions, and profuse nasal discharge and salivation] in 3%, and acne in 15%). Results with elemental iodine were about as effective, but not associated with significant side effects. The most significant side effect with molecular iodine was short-term increased breast pain, which seemed to correspond to a softening of the breast and disappearance of fibrous tissue plaques on physical examination.

The dosage of molecular iodine was 70 to 90 mcg of iodine per kilogram (2.2 pounds) of body weight. This dosage appears to be a safe and effective treatment for FBD. Unfortunately, as of this writing (January 1997) the forms of iodine supplement used in the studies (iodine caseinate and liquid iodine) were not yet available on the marketplace. Kelp may be a suitable alternative in the interim.

Uterine Fibroids

Another common female condition associated with an increased estrogen to progesterone ratio are uterine fibroids—benign growths of the uterus. Fibroids consist of smooth muscle bundles and connective tissue components of the uterus. Uterine fibroids are a relatively common condition; it is estimated that roughly 20% of all women over the age of 30 have uterine fibroids. Fibroids can vary from the size of a pea to that of a grapefruit or larger.

The treatment of uterine fibroids follows the same path as the treatment for PMS and fibrocystic breast disease. For herbal support, I favor using black cohosh. I have had several patients improve dramatically by taking black cohosh (Remifemin) and following the dietary and nutritional supplement guidelines presented in Chapters 7 and 8.

Endometriosis

Endometriosis is a condition in which fragments of the endometrium (the lining of the uterus) are found in other parts of the body. Endometriosis is most prevalent between the ages of 25 and 40 years. It is a common cause of infertility. While the exact cause of endometriosis can vary from patient to patient, most commonly it develops as a result of endometrium fragments traveling up the fallopian tubes and into the pelvic cavity during menses. These displaced fragments of endometrium then respond to the menstrual cycle as if they were still lining the uterus, that is, they bleed. Because the blood cannot escape, it results in the formation of slow-growing cysts, pain, and digestive disturbances.

Treatment of endometriosis short of surgical removal or drugs to stop menstruation is focused at reducing the level of arachidonic acid in the tissue. Arachidonic acid is an omega-6 fatty acid found exclusively in animal foods. In cases of endometriosis, I recommend following a vegetarian diet with the exception of cold-water fish (salmon, mackerel, herring, etc.). I also recommend that the dietary and nutritional supplement guidelines presented in Chapters 7 and 8 be followed. In particular, it is very important to take one tablespoon of high-lignan flaxseed oil daily.

Candidiasis

An overgrowth in the gastrointestinal tract of the usually benign yeast *Candida albicans* is now recognized as a complex medical syndrome known as the *yeast syndrome* or *chronic candidiasis*. The overgrowth of candida is believed to cause a wide variety of symptoms in virtually every system of the body, with the gastrointestinal, genitourinary, endocrine, nervous, and immune systems being the most susceptible. PMS is often linked to chronic candidiasis.

Although chronic candidiasis has been clinically defined for a long time, it was not until Orion Truss published *The Missing Diagnosis* (P.O. Box 26508, Birmingham, AL, 1983) and William Crook published *The Yeast Connection* (Professional Books, 1984) that the public and many physicians became aware of the magnitude of the problem.

The diagnosis of chronic candidiasis is often quite difficult because there is no single specific diagnostic test. Stool cultures and elevated antibody levels to candida are useful diagnostic aids, but they should not be relied upon for diagnosis. The best method for diagnosing chronic candidiasis is a detailed medical history and patient questionnaire. You'll find the questionnaire that I use on page 139.

Candida Questionnaire

Point Score

History

1. Have you taken tetracycline or other antibiotics
   for acne for one month or longer? 25

2. Have you, at any time in your life, taken other
   broad-spectrum antibiotics for respiratory, urinary, or
   other infections for two months or longer, or in short
   courses four or more times in a one-year period? 20

3. Have you ever taken a broad-spectrum antibiotic
   (even a single course)? 6

4. Have you, at any time in your life, been bothered by
   persistent prostatitis, vaginitis, or other problems
   affecting your reproductive organs? 25

5. Have you been pregnant . . .

   One time? 3

   Two or more times? 5

6. Have you taken birth control pills . . .

   For six months to two years? 8

   For more than two years? 15

7. Have you taken prednisone or other cortisone-type
   drugs . . .

   For two weeks or less? 6

   For more than two weeks? 15

8. Does exposure to perfumes, insecticides, fabric
   shop odors, and other chemicals provoke . . .

   Mild symptoms? 5

   Moderate to severe symptoms? 20

9. Are your symptoms worse on damp, muggy days
   or in moldy places? 20

10. Have you had athlete's foot, ringworm, "jock itch,"
    or other chronic infections of the skin or nails?

    Mild to moderate? 10

    Severe or persistent? 20

11. Do you crave sugar? 10

12. Do you crave breads? 10

Continued

Candida Questionnaire *(continued)*

13. Do you crave alcoholic beverages?	10
14. Does tobacco smoke *really* bother you?	10
Total Score of This Section	_____

Major Symptoms

For each of your symptoms, enter the appropriate figure in the Point Score column.

Score column:

> If a symptom is occasional or mild, score 3 points
> If a symptom is frequent and/or moderately severe, score 6 points
> If a symptom is severe and/or disabling, score 9 points

POINT SCORE

1. Fatigue or lethargy _____
2. Feeling of being "drained" _____
3. Poor memory _____
4. Feeling "spacey" or "unreal" _____
5. Depression _____
6. Numbness, burning, or tingling _____
7. Muscle aches _____
8. Muscle weakness or paralysis _____
9. Pain and/or swelling in joints _____
10. Abdominal pain _____
11. Constipation _____
12. Diarrhea _____
13. Bloating _____
14. Persistent vaginal itch _____
15. Persistent vaginal burning _____
16. Prostatitis _____
17. Impotence _____
18. Loss of sexual desire _____
19. Endometriosis _____
20. Cramps and/or other menstrual irregularities _____
21. Premenstrual tension _____

Candida Questionnaire *(continued)*

22. Spots in front of eyes _____

23. Erratic vision _____

Total Score of This Section _____

Other Symptoms

For each of your symptoms, enter the appropriate figure in the Point Score column.

Score column:

If a symptom is occasional or mild, score 1 point
If a symptom is frequent and/or moderately severe, score 2 points
If a symptom is severe and/or disabling, score 3 points

POINT SCORE

1. Drowsiness _____
2. Irritability _____
3. Incoordination _____
4. Inability to concentrate _____
5. Frequent mood swings _____
6. Headache _____
7. Dizziness/loss of balance _____
8. Pressure above ears, feeling of head swelling and tingling _____
9. Itching _____
10. Other rashes _____
11. Heartburn _____
12. Indigestion _____
13. Belching and intestinal gas _____
14. Mucus in stools _____
15. Hemorrhoids _____
16. Dry mouth _____
17. Rash or blisters in mouth _____
18. Bad breath _____
19. Joint swelling or arthritis _____
20. Nasal congestion or discharge _____
21. Postnasal drip _____

Continued

Candida Questionnaire *(continued)*

22. Nasal itching	_____
23. Sore or dry throat	_____
24. Cough	_____
25. Pain or tightness in chest	_____
26. Wheezing or shortness of breath	_____
27. Urinary urgency or frequency	_____
28. Burning on urination	_____
29. Failing vision	_____
30. Burning or tearing of eyes	_____
31. Recurrent infections or fluid in ears	_____
32. Ear pain or deafness	_____
Total Score of This Section	_____
Total Score of All Three Sections	_____

Interpretation

	Women	Men
Yeast-connected health problems are almost certainly present	>180	>140
Yeast-connected health problems are probably present	120–180	90–140
Yeast-connected health problems are possibly present	60–119	40–89
Yeast-connected health problems are less likely present	<60	<40

Adapted from Crook, W. G., *The Yeast Connection*, 2nd ed., Professional Books, Jackson, TN, 1984.

Getting Rid of Candida

Getting rid of candida involves a multifactorial approach designed to address the factors in the intestinal tract (or vaginal tract) that are promoting the excessive growth of the yeast. Here are my primary recommendations if your PMS is related to candida:

1. Get my book *Chronic Candidiasis* (Prima Publishing, 1997) or Dr. Crook's *The Yeast Connection* to educated yourself about candidiasis in greater detail.

2. Eliminate the use of antibiotics, steroids, immune-suppressing drugs, and birth control pills (unless there is absolute medical necessity).

3. Follow these special dietary guidelines:

   Do not eat foods high in sugar.

   Do not eat foods with a high content of yeast or mold including alcoholic beverages, cheeses, dried fruits, melons, and peanuts.

   Do not eat milk and milk products due to their high content of lactose (milk sugar) and trace levels of antibiotics.

4. Avoid all known or suspected allergenic foods.

5. Take a high-potency multiple vitamin and mineral formula (see Chapter 8, page 122).

6. Improve your liver function by taking a lipotropic formula (see Chapter 3, page 23).

7. Ingest 5 to 10 billion viable *L. acidophilus* or *B. bifidum* cells daily (see Chapter 3, page 21).

8. Promote the elimination of candida toxins by taking five grams of a water-soluble fiber source such as guar gum, psyllium seed, or pectin, which can bind to toxins in the gut and promote their excretion at night before retiring.

9. Use nutritional and/or herbal supplements that help control against yeast overgrowth and promote a healthy bacterial flora such as enteric-coated volatile oil preparations (from peppermint, thyme, and/or oregano) at a dosage of 0.2 to 0.4 ml twice daily between meals.

Final Comments

PMS is a syndrome with many different symptoms, therefore, there are a wide range of other situations that are
associated with PMS. This chapter discussed four such situations but there are many others that were touched on
throughout this book, including depression, low thyroid
function, food allergies, corpus luteum insufficiency, and
elevated prolactin levels, as well as other conditions such
as chronic fatigue syndrome, fibromyalgia, and multiple
chemical sensitivity disorder. Successful treatment of PMS
in these cases, obviously, involves improving the underlying situation.

11

Putting It All Together

In order to help you prioritize and implement the measures detailed in the previous chapters of this book, the major steps necessary to effectively treat your PMS are summarized below.

1. Evaluate your PMS symptoms by completing the questionnaire on page 9.

2. Rule out hypothyroidism and depression. Determine your basal body temperature (discussed in Chapter 4, page 31). If your basal body temperature is below 97.8 or if you are suffering from other symptoms associated with PMS, consult your physician for complete thyroid function testing. Determine if depression may be a factor by taking the self-test on page 49. If it is, follow the recommendations given in Chapter 6.

3. Begin following the dietary recommendations given in Chapter 7:

- Follow a vegetarian or predominantly vegetarian diet.
- Reduce your intake of fat.
- Eliminate sugar from your diet.
- Reduce your exposure to environmental estrogens.
- Increase your intake of soy foods.
- Eliminate caffeine.
- Keep your salt intake low.

4. Follow the guidelines for nutritional supplementation in Chapter 8:
- Take a high-quality multiple vitamin and mineral supplement.
- Take additional antioxidants.
- Take one tablespoon of flaxseed oil daily.

5. Select the appropriate herbal support:
- If you have PMS-associated breast pain, infrequent periods, or a history of ovarian cysts take chaste berry extract.
- If you typically experience menstrual cramps, take angelica (dong quai).
- If you are bothered by PMS water retention, take licorice.
- If you suffer from uterine fibroids, take black cohosh extract.

6. Follow the techniques for stress reduction given in Chapter 5.

7. If after at least three complete periods you are not experiencing a significant improvement or complete resolution of symptoms, further support is indicated.

My recommendation is to consult a physician familiar with nutritional therapies for PMS (referral services are given on page 14). The physician should help in identifying possible causative factors and more effective treatment strategies tailored specifically for your case.

References

Chapter 1: An Overview of Premenstrual Syndrome

1. Barnhart KT, Freeman EW, and Sondheimer SJ: A clinician's guide to the premenstrual syndrome. Med Clin North Am 79:1457–72, 1995.

2. Steiner M: Premenstrual dysphoric disorder: An update. Gen Hosp Psychiatry 18:244–50, 1996.

3. Richardson JT: The premenstrual syndrome: A brief history. Soc Sci Med 41:761–7, 1995.

4. Mortola JF: A risk-benefit appraisal of drugs used in the management of premenstrual syndrome. Drug Safety 10:160–9, 1994.

5. Nader S: Premenstrual syndrome. Postgraduate Med 90:173–80, 1991.

6. Smith S: The premenstrual syndrome: Diagnosis and management. Fertility Sterility 53:527–43, 1989.

7. Propping D, Katzorke T, and Belkien L: Diagnosis and therapy of corpus luteum insufficiency in general practice. Therapiwoche 38:2992–3001, 1988.

Chapter 2: PMS Diagnosis and Classifications

1. Smith S: The premenstrual syndrome: Diagnosis and management. Fertility Sterility 53:527–43, 1989.
2. Abraham GE: Nutritional factors in the etiology of the premenstrual tension syndromes. J Reprod Med 28:446–64, 1983.

Chapter 3: The Estrogen to Progesterone Ratio

1. Wang M, et al.: Relationship between symptom severity and steroid variation in women with premenstrual syndrome: Study on serum pregnenolone, pregnenolone sulfate, 5 alpha-pregnane-3, 20-dione and 3 alpha-hydroxy-5 alpha-pregnan-20-one. J Clin Endocrinol 81:1076–82, 1996.
2. Barnhart KT, Freeman EW, and Sondheimer SJ: A clinician's guide to the premenstrual syndrome. Med Clin North Am 79:1457–72, 1995.
3. Facchinetti F, et al.: Oestradiol/progesterone imbalance and the premenstrual syndrome. Lancet 2:1302, 1983.
4. Munday MR, Brush MG, and Taylor RW: Correlations between progesterone, oestradiol and aldosterone levels in the premenstrual syndrome. Clin Endocrinol 14:1–9, 1981.
5. Backstrom T and Mattson B: Correlation of symptoms in premenstrual tension to oestrogen and progesterone concentrations in blood plasma. Neuropsychobiol 1:80–6, 1975.
6. Reid RL: PMS etiology: Medical theories. In: Gynecology: Essentials of Clinical Practice. Keye WR Jr (ed.). WB Saunders, Philadelphia, 1988, pp.66–93.
7. Biskind MS and Biskind GR: Diminution in ability of the liver to inactivate estrogen in vitamin B complex deficiency. Science 94:462, 1941.
8. Biskind MS: Nutritional deficiency in the etiology of menorrhagia, metrorrhagia, cystic mastitis and premenstrual tension: Treatment with vitamin B complex. J Clin Endo Met 3:227–34, 1943.
9. Chuong CJ, Hsi BP and Gibbons WE: Periovulatory beta-endorphin levels in premenstrual syndrome. Obstet Gynecol 83:755–60, 1995.

10. Wynn V, et al.: Tryptophan, depression and steroidal contraception. J Steroid Biochem 6:965–70, 1975.

11. Bermond P: Therapy of side effects of oral contraceptive agents with vitamin B6. Acta Vitaminol-Enzymol 4:45–54, 1982.

12. Halbreich U, et al.: Serum-prolactin in women with premenstrual syndrome. Lancet 2:654–6, 1976.

13. O'Brien PM and Symonds EM: Prolactin levels in the premenstrual syndrome. Br J Obst Gyn 89:306–8, 1982.

14. Goldin B and Gorsbach S: The effect of milk and lactobacillus feeding on human intestinal bacterial enzyme activity. Am J Clin Nutr 39:756–61, 1984.

15. Hughes VL and Hillier SL: Microbiologic characteristics of lactobacillus products used for colonization of the vagina. Obstet Gynecol 75:244–8, 1990.

16. Freeman E, et al.: Ineffectiveness of progesterone suppository treatment for premenstrual syndrome. JAMA 264:349–53, 1990.

17. Maddocks S, et al.: A double-blind placebo-controlled trial of progesterone vaginal suppositories in the treatment of premenstrual syndrome. Am J Obstet Gynecol 154:573–81, 1986.

18. Andersch B and Hahn LJ: Progesterone treatment of premenstrual tension: A double blind study. Psychosom Res 29:489–93, 1985.

19. Dennerstein L, et al.: Progesterone and the premenstrual syndrome: A double blind crossover trial. Br Med J 290:1617–21, 1985.

20. Baker ER, et al.: Efficacy of progesterone vaginal suppositories in alleviation of nervous symptoms in patients with premenstrual syndrome. J Assist Reprod Genet 12(3):205–9, 1995.

21. Magill PJ: Investigation of the efficacy of progesterone pessaries in the relief of symptoms of premenstrual syndrome: Progesterone Study Group. Br J Gen Pract 45(400):589–93, 1995.

Chapter 4: Low Thyroid Function in PMS

1. Brayshaw ND and Brayshaw DD: Thyroid hypofunction in premenstrual syndrome. New Engl J Med 315:1486–7, 1986.

2. Roy-Byrne PP, et al.: TSH and prolactin responses to TRH in patients with premenstrual syndrome. Am J Psychiatry 144:480–4, 1987.

3. Girdler SS, Pedersen CA, and Light KC: Thyroid axis function during the menstrual cycle in women with premenstrual syndrome. Psychoneuroendocrin 20:395–403, 1995.

4. Schmidt PJ, et al.: Thyroid function in women with premenstrual syndrome. J Clin Endocrinol Metab 76:671–4, 1993.

5. Althaus U, Staub JJ, Ryff-De Leche A, et al.: LDL/HDL-changes in subclinial hypothyroidism: Possible risk factors for coronary heart disease. Clin Endocrinol 28:157-63, 1988.

6. Dean JW and Fowler PBS: Exaggerated responsiveness to thyrotrophin releasing hormone: A risk factor in women with artery disease. Br Med J 290:1555–61, 1985.

7. Turnbridge WMG, Evered DC, and Hall R: Lipid profiles and cardiovascular disease in the Wickham area with particular reference to thyroid failure. Clin Endocrinol 7:495–508, 1977.

8. Gold M, Pottash A, and Extein I: Hypothyroidism and depression: Evidence from complete thyroid function evaluation. JAMA 245:1919–22, 1981.

9. Joffe R, Roy-Byrne P, and Udhe T: Thyroid function and affective illness: A reappraisal. Biol Psychiatry 19:1685–91, 1984.

10. Krupsky M, et al.: Musculoskeletal symptoms as a presenting sign of long-standing hypothyroidism. Isr J Med Sci 23:1110–3, 1987.

11. Hochberg MC, et al.: Hypothyroidism presenting as a polymyositis-like syndrome. Arthr Rheum 19:1363–6, 1976.

12. Barnes BO and Galton L: Hypothyroidism: The Unsuspected Illness. Thomas Crowell, New York, 1976.

13. Langer SE and Scheer JF: Solved: The Riddle of Illness. Keats, New Canaan, CT, 1984.

14. Jennings IW: Vitamins in Endocrine Metabolism. C.C. Thomas, Springfield, IL, 1970.

15. Prasad A: Clinical, biochemical and nutritional spectrum of zinc deficiency in human subjects: An update. Ntr Rev 41:197–208, 1983.

16. Lennon D, Nagle F, Stratman F, et al.: Diet and exercise training effects on resting metabolic rate. Int J Obesity 9:39–47, 1985.

Chapter 5: Stress, Endorphins, and Exercise

1. Holmes TH and Rahe RH: The social readjustment scale. J Psychosomatic Res 11:213–8, 1967.

2. Carroll BJ, Curtis GC, and Mendels J: Cerebrospinal fluid and plasma-free cortisol concentrations in depression. Psychol Med 6:235–44, 1976.

3. Facchinetti F, et al.: Changes of opioid modulation of the hypothalamo-pituitary axis in patients with severe premenstrual syndrome. Psychosomatic Med 56:418–22, 1994.

4. Altar C, et al.: Glucocorticoid induction of tryptophan oxygenase. Biochem Pharmacol 32:979–84, 1983.

5. Aganoff JA and Boyle GJ: Aerobic exercise, mood states and menstrual cycle symptoms. J Psychosom Res 38:183–92, 1994.

6. Choi PY and Salmon P: Symptom changes across the menstrual cycle in competitive sportswomen, exercisers and sedentary women. Br J Clin Psychol 34:447–60, 1995.

7. Steege JF and Blumenthal JA: The effects of aerobic exercise on premenstrual symptoms in middle-aged women: A preliminary study. J Psychosom Res 37(2):127–33, 1993.

8. Weyerer S and Kupfer B: Physical exercise and psychological health. Sports Med 17:108–16, 1994.

9. Byrne A and Byrne DG: The effect of exercise on depression, anxiety and other mood states: A review. J Psychosom Res 37:565–74, 1993.

10. Dua J and Hargreaves L: Effect of aerobic exercise on negative affect, positive affect, stress, and depression. Percept Mot Skills 75:355–61, 1992.

11. Stein PN and Motta RW: Effects of aerobic and nonaerobic exercise on depression and self-concept. Percept Mot Skills 74:79–89, 1992.

12. Casper RC: Exercise and mood. World Rev Nutr Diet 71:115–43, 1993.

13. LaFontaine TP, et al.: Aerobic exercise and mood: A brief review, 1985–1990. Sports Med 13:160–70, 1992.

14. Lobstein D, Mosbacher BJ, and Ismail AH: Depression as a powerful discriminator between physically active and sedentary middle-aged men. J Psychosom Res 27:69–76, 1983.

15. Kuczmierczyk AR, Johnson CC, and Labrum AH: Coping styles in women with premenstrual syndrome. Acta Psychiatr Scand 89:301–5, 1994.

16. Van Zak DB, et al.: Biofeedback treatments for premenstrual and premenstrual affective syndromes. Int J Psychosom 41:53–60, 1994.

17. Kirkby RJ: Changes in premenstrual symptoms and irrational thinking following cognitive-behavioral coping skills training. J Consult Clin Psychol 62:1026–32, 1994.

Chapter 6: Depression, Low Levels of Serotonin, and PMS

1. Barnhart KT, Freeman EW, and Sondheimer SJ: A clinician's guide to the premenstrual syndrome. Med Clin North Am 79:1457–72, 1995.

2. Eriksson E, et al.: Cerebrospinal fluid levels of monoamine metabolites: A preliminary study of their relation to menstrual cycle phase, sex steroids, and pituitary hormones in healthy women and in women with premenstrual syndrome. Neuropsychopharmacol 11:201–13, 1994.

3. Halbreich U, et al.: Low plasma gamma-aminobutyric acid levels during the late luteal phase of women with premenstrual dysphoric disorder. Am J Psychiatry 153(5):718–20, 1996.

4. Thiede HM and Walper A: Inhibition of MAO and COMT by hypericum extracts and hypericin. J Geriatr Psychiatry Neurol 7(Suppl 1):S54–6, 1994.

5. Thiele B, Brink I, and Ploch M: Modulation of cytokine expression by hypericum extract. J Geriatr Psychiatry Neurol 7(Suppl 1):S60–2, 1994.

6. Perovic S and Muller WEG: Pharmacological profile of hypericum extract: Effect of serotonin uptake by postsynaptic receptors. Arzneim Forsch 45:1145–8, 1995.

7. Linde K, et al.: St. John's wort for depression: An overview and meta-analysis of randomised clinical trials. Br Med J 313:253–8, 1996.

8. Pande AC and Sayler ME: Adverse events and treatment discontinuations in fluoxetine clinical trials. Int J Psychopharmacol 8:267–9, 1993.

9. Balon R, et al.: Sexual dysfunction during antidepressant treatment. J Clin Psychiatry 54:209–12, 1993; Herman M and Goldbloom DS: Fluoxetine-induced sexual dysfunction. J Clin Psychiatry 42:25–7, 1990.

10. Woelk H, Burkard G, and Grunwald J: Benefits and risks of the hypericum extract LI 160: Drug monitoring study with 3250 patients. J Geriatr Psychiatry Neurol 7(Suppl 1):S34–8, 1994.

11. Jarrett RB and Rush AJ: Short-term psychotherapy of depressive disorders: Current status and future directions. Psychiatry 57:115–32, 1994.

12. Robins CJ and Hayes AM: An appraisal of cognitive therapy. J Consult Clin Psychol 61:205–14, 1993.

13. Evans M, et al.: Differential relapse following cognitive therapy and pharmacotherapy for depression. Arch Gen Psychiatry 49:802–8, 1992.

Chapter 7: Dietary Guidelines

1. Abraham GE: Nutritional factors in the etiology of the premenstrual tension syndromes. J Reprod Med 28:446–64, 1983.

2. Gorbach SL and Goldin BR: Diet and the excretion and enterohepatic cycling of estrogens. Prev Med 16:525–31, 1987.

3. Goldin BR, et al.: Estrogen patterns and plasma levels in vegetarian and omnivorous women. New Engl J Med 307:1542–7, 1982.

4. National Research Council: Diet and Health: Implications for Reducing Chronic Disease Risk. National Academy Press, Washington, D.C., 1989.

5. Kohlmeier L and Hastings SB: Epidemiologic evidence of a role of carotenoids in cardiovascular disease prevention. Am J Clin Nutr 62(Suppl.):1370S–6S, 1995.

6. Longcope C, et al.: The effect of a low fat diet on oestrogen metabolism. J Clin Endocrinol Metab 64:1246–50, 1987.

7. Woods MN, et al.: Low-fat, high-fiber diet and serum estrone sulfate in premenopausal women. Am J Clin Nutr 49:1179–83, 1989.

8. Jones DY: Influence of dietary fat on self-reported menstrual symptoms. Physiol Behav 40:483-7, 1987.

9. Longnecker MP: Do trans fatty acids in margarine and other foods increase the risk of coronary heart disease? Epidemiology 4:492-5, 1993.

10. Rossignol AM and Bonnlander H: Prevalence and severity of the premenstrual syndrome: Effects of foods and beverages that are sweet or high in sugar content. J Reprod Med 36:131-6, 1991.

11. Yudkin J and Eisa O: Dietary sucrose and oestradiol concentration in young men. Ann Nutr Metabol 32:53-5, 1988.

12. Falck F, et al.: Pesticides and polychlorinated biphenyl residues in human breast lipids and their relation to breast cancer. Archives of Environ Health 47:143-6, 1992.

13. Sharpe RM and Skakkebaek NE: Are oestrogens involved in falling sperm counts and disorders of the male reproduction tract? Lancet 341:1392-5, 1993.

14. Mott L and Broad M: Pesticides in Food. Natural Resources Defense Council, San Francisco, 1984.

15. Quillin P: Safe Eating. Evans, New York, 1990.

16. Messina M and Barnes S: The roles of soy products in reducing risk of cancer. J Natl Cancer Inst 83:541-6, 1991.

17. Messina M and Messina V: Increasing the use of soy foods and their potential role in cancer prevention. J Am Diet Assoc 91:836-40, 1991.

18. Rossignol AM and Bonnlander H: Caffeine-containing beverages, total fluid consumption, and premenstrual syndrome. Am J Public Health 80:1106-10, 1990.

19. Rossignol AM: Caffeine-containing beverages and premenstrual syndrome in young women. Am J Public Health 75:1335-7, 1985.

20. Kreitsch K, et al.: Prevalence, presenting symptoms, and psychological characteristics of individuals experiencing a diet-related mood disturbance. Behav Ther 19:593-4, 1985.

21. Christensen L: Psychological distress and diet: Effects of sucrose and caffeine. J Apl Nutr 40:44-50, 1988.

22. Stanto JL and Keast DR: Serum cholesterol, fat intake, and breakfast consumption in the United States adult population. J Am Coll Nutr 8:567-72, 1989.

Chapter 8: Nutritional Supplementation

1. Berman MK, et al.: Vitamin B6 in premenstrual syndrome. J Am Diet Assoc 90:859–61, 1990.

2. Kliejnen J, Ter Riet G, and Knipschild P: Vitamin B6 in the treatment of premenstrual syndrome: A review. Br J Obstet Gynaecol 97:847–52, 1990.

3. Barr W: Pyridoxine supplements in the premenstrual syndrome. Practitioner 228:425–7, 1984.

4. Zempleni J: Pharmacokinetics of vitamin B6 supplements in humans. J Am Coll Nutr 14:579–86, 1995.

5. Cohen M and Bendich A: Safety of pyridoxine: A review of human and animal studies. Toxicol Letters 34:129–39, 1986.

6. Parry GJ and Bredesen DE: Sensory neuropathy with low-dose pyridoxine. Neurol 35:1466–8, 1985.

7. Waterston JA and Gilligan BS: Pyridoxine neuropathy. Med J Aust 146:640–2, 1987.

8. Majumdar P and Boylan M: Alteration of tissue magnesium levels in rats by dietary vitamin B6 supplementation. Int J Vitamin Nutr Res 59:300–3, 1989.

9. Posacki C, et al.: Plasma copper, zinc, and magnesium levels in patients with premenstrual tension syndrome. Acta Obstet Gynecol Scand 73:452–5, 1994.

10. Abraham GE: Nutritional factors in the etiology of the premenstrual tension syndromes. J Repro Med 28:446–64, 1983.

11. Piesse JW: Nutritional factors in the premenstrual syndrome. Int Clin Nutr Rev 4:54–81, 1984.

12. Facchinetti F, et al.: Oral magnesium successfully relieves premenstrual mood changes. Obstet Gynecol 78:177–81, 1991.

13. Rosenstein DL, et al.: Magnesium measures across the menstrual cycle in premenstrual syndrome. Biol Psychiatr 35:557–61, 1994.

14. London RS, Bradley R, and Chiamori NY: Effect of a nutritional supplement on premenstrual symptomatology in women with premenstrual syndrome: A double-blind longitudinal study. J Am Coll Nutr 10:494–9, 1991.

15. Stewart A: Clinical and biochemical effects of nutritional supplementation on the premenstrual syndrome. J Reprod Med 32:435–41, 1987.

16. Lindberg JS, et al.: Magnesium bioavailability from magnesium citrate and magnesium oxide. J Am Coll Nutr 9:48–55, 1990.

17. Bohmer T, et al.: Bioavailability of oral magnesium supplementation in female students evaluated from elimination of magnesium in 24-hour urine. Magnesium Trace Elem 9:272–8, 1990.

18. Penland JG and Johnson PE: Dietary calcium and manganese effects on menstrual cycle symptoms. Am J Obstet Gynecol 168:1417–23, 1993.

19. Thys-Jacob S, et al.: Calcium supplementation in premenstrual syndrome: A randomized crossover trial. J Gen Intern Med 4:183–9, 1989.

20. Thys-Jacobs S, et al.: Reduced bone mass in women with premenstrual syndrome. J Women Health 4:161–8, 1995.

21. Chuong CJ and Dawson EB: Zinc and copper levels in premenstrual syndrome. Fertility Sterility 62:313–20, 1994.

22. Judd AM, Macleod RM, and Login IS: Zinc acutely, selectively and reversibly inhibits pituitary prolactin secretion. Brain Res 294:190–2, 1984.

23. London RS, et al: The effect of alpha-tocopherol on premenstrual symptomatology: A double-blind study. II: Endocrine correlates. J Am Col Nutr 3:351–6, 1984.

24. Horrobin DF, et al.: Abnormalities in plasma essential fatty acid levels in women with premenstrual syndrome and with non-malignant breast disease. J Nutr Med 2:259–64, 1991.

25. Erasmus U: Fats That Heal, Fats That Kill. Alive Books, Burnaby, B.C., Canada, 1995.

26. Budeiri D, et al.: Is evening primrose oil of value in the treatment of premenstrual syndrome? Control Clin Trials 17:60–8, 1996.

27. Khoo SK, Munro C, and Battistutta D: Evening primrose oil and treatment of premenstrual syndrome. Med J Austral 153:189–92, 1990.

28. Cerin A, et al.: Hormonal and biochemical profiles of premenstrual syndrome: Treatment with essential fatty acids. Acta Obstet Gynecol Scand 72:337–43, 1993.

29. Collins A, et al.: Essential fatty acids in the treatment of premenstrual syndrome. Acta Obstet Gynecol 81:93–8, 1993.

30. Serraino M and Thompson LU: The effect of flaxseed on early risk markers for mammary carcinogenesis. Cancer Letters 60:135–42, 1991.

31. Serraino M and Thompson LU: Flaxseed supplementation and early markers of colon carcinogenesis. Cancer Letters 63:159–65, 1992.

32. Serraino M and Thompson LU: The effect of flaxseed supplementation on the initiation and promotional stages of mammary tumorigenesis. Nutr Cancer 17:153–9, 1992.

33. Thompson LU, et al.: Mammalian lignan production from various foods. Nutr Cancer 16:43–52, 1991.

34. Adlercreutz H, et al.: Determination of urinary lignans and phytoestrogen metabolites, potential antiestrogens and anticarcinogens in urine of women in various habitual diets. J Steroid Biochem 25:791–7, 1986.

35. Bougnoix P, et al.: Alpha-linolenic acid content of adipose breast tissue: A host determinant of the risk of early metastasis in breast cancer. Br J Cancer 70:330–4, 1994.

36. Rose DP and Hatala MA: Dietary fatty acids and breast cancer invasion and metastasis. Nutr Cancer 21:103–11, 1994.

Chapter 9: Herbal Support for PMS

1. Harada M, Suzuki M, and Ozaki Y: Effect of Japanese angelica root and peony root on uterine contraction in the rabbit in situ. J Pharm Dyn 7:304–11, 1984.

2. Yoshiro K: The physiological actions of tang-kuei and cnidium. Bull Oriental Healing Arts Inst USA 10:269–78, 1985.

3. Costello CH and Lynn EV: Estrogenic substances from plants: I. Glycyrrhiza. J Am Pharm Soc 39:177–80, 1950.

4. Kumagai A, Nishino K, Shimomura A, Kin T, and Yamamura Y: Effect of glycyrrhizin on estrogen action. Endocrinol Japon 14:34–8, 1967.

5. Farese RV, et al.: Licorice-induced hypermineralocorticoidism. N Engl J Med 325:1223–7, 1991.

6. Stormer FC, Reistad R, and Alexander J: Glycyrrhizic acid in licorice: Evaluation of health hazard. Fd Chem Toxicol 31:303–12, 1993.

7. Baron J, et al.: Metabolic studies, aldosterone secretion rate and plasma renin after carbonoxolone sodium as biogastrone. Br Med J 2:793–5, 1969.

8. Duker EM, et al.: Effects of extracts from *Cimicifuga racemosa* on gonadotropin release in menopausal women and ovariectomized rats. Planta Medica 57:420–4, 1991.

9. Stolze H: An alternative to treat menopausal complaints. Gyne 3:14–6, 1982.

10. Warnecke G: Influencing menopausal symptoms with a phytotherapeutic agent. Med Welt 36:871–4, 1985.

11. Stoll W: Phytopharmacon influences atrophic vaginal epithelium: Double-blind study—*Cimicifuga* vs. estrogenic substances. Therapeuticum 1:23–31, 1986.

12. Schildge E: Essay on the treatment of premenstrual and moenopausal mood swings and depressive states. Rigelh Biol Umsch 19(2):18–22, 1964.

13. Dittmar FW, et al.: Premenstrual syndrome: Treatment with a phytopharmaceutical. Therapiewoche Gynakol 5:60–8, 1992.

14. Peteres-Welte C and Albrecht M: Menstrual abnormalities and PMS: *Vitex agnus-castus.* Therapiewoche Gynakol 7:49–52, 1994.

15. Milewicz A, et al.: *Vitex agnus-castus* in the treatment of luteal phase defects due to hyperprolactinemia. 43:752–6, 1993.

Chapter 10: Other Female Conditions Associated with PMS

1. Cole EN, Sellwood RA, England PG, and Griffiths K: Serum prolactin concentrations in benign breast disease throughout the menstrual cycle. J Cancer 13:597–603, 1977.

2. Peters F, Schuth W, Scheurich B, and Breckwoldt M: Serum prolactin levels in patients with fibrocystic breast disease. Obstet Gynecol 64:381–5, 1984.

3. Boyle CA, Berkowitz GS, LiVolsi VA, et al.: Caffeine consumption and fibrocystic breast disease: A case-control epidemiologic study. JNCI 72:1015–9, 1984.

4. Minton JP, Abou-Issa H, Reiches N, and Roseman JM: Clinical and biochemical studies on methylxanthine-related fibrocystic breast disease. Surgery 90:299–304, 1981.

5. Minton JP, Foecking MK, Webster DJT, and Matthews RH: Caffeine, cyclic nucleotides, and breast disease. Surgery 86:105–9, 1979.

6. Ernster VL, Mason L, Goodson WH, et al: Effects of caffeine-free diet on benign breast disease: A random trial. Surgery 91:263–7, 1982.

7. Welsh C, Scieska K, Senn E, and Dehoog J: Caffeine (1,3,7-trimethylxanthine) a temperate promoter of DMBA-induced rat mammary gland carcinogenesis. Int J Ca 32:479–83, 1983.

8. Estes NC: Mastodynia due to fibrocystic disease of the breast controlled with thyroid hormone. A J Surg 142:764–6, 1981.

9. Ghent WR, et al.: Iodine replacement in fibrocystic disease of the breast. Can J Surg 36:453–60, 1993.

Index

C

Caffeine
    content of drinks, 76
    eliminating, 75–76
    fibrocystic breast disease and,
        75, 134–135
Calcium, 111–112
Calories
    exchange recommendation
        examples, 82–85
    requirement, 80–81
Cancer
    alpha-linolenic acid and, 120
    flaxseed oil benefits, 117–120
Candidiasis, 138–143
    overview, 138
    questionnaire, 139–142
    treatment, 142–143
Carbohydrate craving in PMS-C, 8
Carbohydrates, complex, 79–80,
        90–92
Carotenes, 63–64, 123
Causal factors
    classification by, 10–13
    detecting, 11–13
    fibrocystic breast disease, 134
    overview, 5–6, 11
Center for Epidemilogical Studies-
        Depression test, 47–48,
        49–51
Cereals. *See* Grains
CES-D test, 47–48, 49–51
Chaste berry
    dosage, 24, 130
    overview, 129–130
    prolactin levels and, 19–20
Cheese. *See* Dairy products
Chelation, 110
Cholestasis, 16–17
Cholesterol, 62, 63, 96
Chronic candidiasis. *See* Candidi-
        asis
Chronic Candidiasis, 143
Cimicifuga racemosa (black
        cohosh), 128–129
Classifications of PMS
    Abraham's system, 7–10
    by causative factors, 10–13
Coffee, 76
Cognitive therapy, 45, 58–59
Commission E, 52–53
Complete protein, 93
Complex carbohydrates, 79–80,
        90–92

Coping strategies, 43–44
Corpus luteum insufficiency, 5
Corticosteroids, 36, 38
Corticotropin-releasing hormone
        (CRH), 38
Cortisol
    assessing level of, 38
    elevated levels, 38–39
    function of, 36
Creams, progesterone, 25–26
CRH stimulation test, 38
Crook, William, 138

D

Dairy products
    candidiasis and, 143
    Exchange lists, 98, 99–100
    fat content, 69
    milk, 98
Dehydroepiandrosterone (DHEA),
        38
Depression, 47–59
    antidepressant drugs, 45, 47
    biogenic amine hypothesis, 48,
        51
    elevated cortisol levels and,
        38–39
    estrogen excess and, 17–18
    exercise and, 41–42
    natural treatment of, 57–58
    in PMS-D, 10
    PMS treatment and, 145
    psychotherapy for, 44–45, 58–59
    St. John's wort extract for,
        52–57
    test for, 47–48, 49–51
DHEA (dehydroepiandrosterone),
        38
Diabetes and fruit juices, 88
Diagnosis. *See also* Tests
    adrenal function assessment,
        38
    candidiasis, 138–142
    of hypothyroidism, 28, 30–32
    self-diagnosis, vi
Diagnos-Techs, 24, 38
Diet, 61–104. *See also* Exchange
        System
    caffeine, eliminating, 75–76
    for candidiasis, 143
    cholesterol, 62, 63
    elimination diet, 103–104
    environmental estrogens,
        avoiding, 70–73

prevalence of, 133
treatment, 134–136
Fibroids, uterine, 137
Fish. *See* Meat and fish
Flatulence and legumes, 93–94
Flavonoids, 63, 64
Flax for Life, 96
Flaxseed oil
    alpha-linolenic acid in, 120
    anticancer benefits, 117–120
    Basil Dressing, 96
    daily supplementation, 124
    as GLA supplement, 117
    lignans in, 119–120
Food allergies, 102–104
Frame size determination, 80–81
Fruits. *See* Produce

G
GABA (gamma-aminobutyric acid), 47, 48
Gallstones, 17
Gamma-aminobutyric acid (GABA), 47, 48
Gamma-linolenic acid (GLA), 116–117
Gastrointestinal flora, 20–22, 64
GLA (gamma-linolenic acid), 116–117
Glucocorticoids, 36
Glycyrrhiza glabra (licorice root), 127–128
Goitrogens, 34
Grains
    dietary fiber in, 66
    Exchange list, 90–92
    fat content, 69
    overview, 90–91
    sprouting, 94–95
Great Smokies Diagnostic Laboratory, 24

H
Halogenated hydrocarbons, 70–73
Healing Power of Foods, The, 79
Healthy Exchange System. See Exchange System
Height and weight table, 81
HerbalGram, 53
Herbs, 125–131
    angelica (dong quai), 126–127
    black cohosh, 128–129
    for candidiasis, 143
    combining, 130–131
    for estrogen excess, 24

German knowledge of, 52–53
licorice root, 127–128
overview, 125–126
prolactin levels and, 19–20
recommendations, 146
St. John's wort extract, 52–57
Holmes, T. H., 35
Homeostasis, 124
Hormones. *See also* Estrogen; Progesterone
    hypothyroidism symptoms, 29
    in normal menstrual cycle, 2–4
    patterns in PMS, 4–5
Hydrogenated oils, 67
Hyperhydration in PMS-H, 10
Hypericum perforatum. See St. John's wort extract
Hypothalamus, 2–3
Hypothyroidism, 27–34
    diagnosing, 30–32
    exercise and, 34
    fibrocystic breast disease and, 135–136
    importance of diagnosing, 28
    nutritional support, 33–34
    PMS treatment and, 145
    prevalence of, 27–28
    symptoms, 28–30
    treatment, 32–34

I, J
Iodides, 136
Iodine, 33–34, 135–136
Irritability, psychotherapy for, 58–59

K
17-Ketosteroids, 36, 38
Krebs cycle, 110

L
Laboratories
    for adrenal stress index, 38
    for ELISA tests, 104
    for liver detoxification profile, 24
    progesterone level monitoring, 26
Lactobacillus acidophilus, 21–22
Legumes, 92–95
    cooking dried legumes, 94
    dietary fiber in, 66
    Exchange list, 95
    fat content, 68
    flatulence and, 93–94